HEALTHWISE HANDBOOK

HEALTHWISE HANDBOOK

Toni M. Roberts

Kathleen McIntosh Tinker

Donald W. Kemper

A DOLPHIN BOOK
Doubleday & Company, Inc.
GARDEN CITY, NEW YORK   1979

This book was originally funded and published by Healthwise, Incorporated, 111 South Sixth Street, Boise, Idaho 83702.

The self-care guidelines in this book are based on the combined research and recommendation of responsible medical sources and have been reviewed by numerous physicians, nurses, and other health professionals for accuracy and safety. The authors and publishers, however, disclaim any responsibility for any adverse effects or consequences resulting from the misapplication or injudicious use of any of the material contained herein.

Library of Congress Cataloging in Publication Data

Roberts, Toni M
    Healthwise handbook.

    Includes index.
    1. Medicine, Popular.   2. Health.   I. Tinker,
Kathleen McIntosh, joint author.   II. Kemper, Donald W.,
joint author.   III. Title.
RC81.R663   616'.024
ISBN: 0-385-14339-7
Library of Congress Catalog Card Number 78–55852

The preparation and publication of this handbook has been assisted by the W. K. Kellogg Foundation of Battle Creek, Michigan.

Contents

Note

Healthwise, Incorporated is a nonprofit organization dedicated to helping people accept greater responsibility for their health. In addition to
this handbook, Healthwise has developed videotapes and other instruc-
tional aids useful for supporting workshops or classes in medical self-
care. Individuals, clinics and other organizations wishing information
about sponsoring self-care workshops should contact Healthwise directly at 111 South Sixth Street, Boise, Idaho 83702.

Foreword

This handbook is designed to help guide your decisions about common health problems. Although much effort was made to base the handbook's guidelines on careful research and professional concensus, they will not always be right for your situation.

Health problems are in some ways unique to each individual. These individual differences must be considered if the book is to be used wisely.

This book does not eliminate the lay person's need for professional medical help. Instead it should strengthen the communication and partnership between patient and professional.

Use this handbook as a tool for improving health care decisions. Should you receive professional advice in conflict with this book heed the health professional; your individual history and circumstances can then be taken into account. Should recommended self-care of any problem fail to provide positive results within a reasonable period, you should consult a health professional.

Acknowledgments

Many individuals have reviewed, critiqued, corrected, and edited the editions of this handbook. We are indebted to all of them for their commitment and enthusiasm in accepting the seemingly endless procession of drafts.

Our deepest thanks to: Carolyn Rapp, Rick Sager, and Phyllis Salter, members of our Board of Directors who gave us direction and shared many practical insights; Bob Matthies, M.D., a physician long committed to consumer education who cheerfully gave many many hours; staff at Gem Health Association, notably Patricia Powell and Bruce Moody, M.D.; staff of the Central District Health Department, particularly Marsha Irvin, Public Health Nutritionist, and Karen Slusser, Dental Hygienist, who have willingly and wisely advised us.

Our thanks, too, to the many local health professionals whose reviews and comments added greatly to the quality and completeness of the handbook: Paul Creighton, M.D., Joseph Daglan, M.D., L. J. Fagnan, M.D., Scott Freeman, D.M.D., Mike Gibson, M.D., Bob Gudmundsen, D.M.D., Sharon Job, R.N., Dave Johnson, M.D., Beverly Ludders, M.D., Ed Matthes, D.M.D., Judy Peterson, Public Health Nutritionist John Rawlings, R.Ph., Dick Starkey, M.D., Virginia Turner, R.Ph., and the many others who commented a lot or a little. Thanks, too, to Diane Barbosa and Judy Fuller for their distinct viewpoints.

A good deal of the inspiration and some of the most practical health tips for the *Healthwise Handbook* came from Keith Sehnert, M.D., who pioneered the concept of "the activated patient." Good ideas for some changes in the second edition came from Don Vickery, M.D.

We added a chapter on mental wellness to this edition, and lots of good people helped us on that challenging task. First, thanks to Francis Kirk and H. A. P. Myers, M.D., whose ideas formed the basic framework of the chapter. Thanks, too, to the reviewers: Michael Eisenbeiss, Tom Ferguson, M.D., David Goodenough, Susan Gunn, Ph.D., Donna Ilett, Mark Mays, Ph.D., Cathy Morris, June Perry, Martin Seidenfeld, Ph.D., and Colin Wright.

Program development funds for the *Healthwise Handbook* were provided under a grant from the W. K. Kellogg Foundation of Battle Creek, Michigan.

Finally, we want to acknowledge the almost superhuman efforts of Elizabeth Martin in typing and laying out the first edition of the *Healthwise Handbook,* and we thank Annie Cary-Engel, who joined the team in time to give us lots of help on this second edition.

Introduction

We wrote this handbook because we believe each individual is responsible for his or her own health. We hope it will help you assume that responsibility in maintaining and improving family health. You can save time, worry, and needless expense by knowing when to treat minor illnesses at home and how to recognize when more skilled care is needed. This handbook can help you make those decisions.

You are the person best qualified to keep yourself healthy and know when you or someone in your family is ill. You know yourself and your family better than anyone else. With a little practice, you can learn what is normal and quickly recognize when something is not. Combining your skills and efforts with those of your health professional will create a health care team far more effective than either one working alone.

This book can best help you become responsible for family health if you read it, and then use it as a handy reference to health problems.

Here's a brief outline of what you'll find:

Chapter 1 "Home Physical Examinations"—How to give a home exam to establish a basis for evaluating problems. What to look for to learn what's normal for each family member and recognize symptoms of illness when they occur. How to get the most from a visit to your doctor.

Chapters 2–8 Descriptions of many common health problems— how to recognize and treat them, and suggestions of when to get professional care.

Chapter 9 "Dental Care"—Why you don't have to lose your teeth, and how to save them.

Chapter 10 "Eating Wisely"—A brief look at nutrition and how to help your family establish good eating habits.

Chapter 11 "Mental Wellness"— How to promote and maintain good mental health.

Chapter 12 "Becoming Healthwise"—What *you* do, day in and day out, controls how long you'll live much more than what a doctor does *for* you. A look at how you can change your lifestyle to improve well-being and possibly extend your life.

Chapter 13 "Your Home Health Center"—Practical advice on health tools for the healthwise person.

Chapter 14 "Your Medicine Chest"—A look at some useful drugs for relief of common symptoms. Advice on drug therapy and some cautions about our instant cure oriented society.

Chapter 15 "Family Medical Records"—A place to establish organized family medical records. Here are sample forms for recording the information gained in home physicals, health histories, immunization records, medical allergies, and other information about your family's health.

Being healthwise means knowing how to maintain your health and well-being and knowing what to do when faced with minor illness. It means being able to discuss your health problems with health professionals and reaching good solutions together. We can't promise that one reading of this handbook will make you healthwise. But it should help you relax and feel more confident as you take responsibility for that most precious commodity—your family's health.

1

Home Physical Examinations

THE IMPORTANCE OF HOME PHYSICALS

Home physical examinations are the first step in taking responsibility for family health. You are the person who knows your family best: good home physicals help you learn what's normal for each family member so you can recognize a problem when it arises.

This chapter outlines the steps in a home physical exam. Completing an exam is fun and easy, and shouldn't take more than half an hour. Children learn to view an exam as an expression of your love, so that the home exam creates a perfect atmosphere for introducing good health practices to your children, practices that may become life-long habits.

Plan to complete a thorough home physical of each family member twice a year. Because infants and young children grow and change so quickly, they need more frequent exams. A complete check every month and a quick once-over at bath time is best for them. As children grow, they will want to do parts of the physical for themselves, which is fine as long as good records are maintained.

The home physical isn't only for routine check-ups. When someone becomes ill, complete an exam and compare the results to a physical given when the person was well. Record all your physicals on the Home Physical Exam form found in "Family Medical Records," page 231. You need good clear written records, for no one can remember everything.

The physical exam described in this chapter is generally for young children. The exam is just about the same for older children, infants, or adults, with some changes as noted.

BEFORE THE EXAM

Home physicals will be easier if

you follow the same routine each time. Do the exam in a comfortable, well-lighted room where interruptions will be limited. Exams should be pleasant experiences. You can help by not being rigid about the exam. Whether your child lies down or sits for the exam isn't important. A toy or one of your tools may divert a nervous child, and be sure you warm your hands before touching your patient.

Then relax and have confidence. Your attitude will surely affect the person you are examining.

TOOLS YOU'LL NEED

Doing a good, thorough home physical exam requires only a few tools:

- a penlight or flashlight
- an accurate thermometer
- some kind of tongue depressor. Some people like clean popsicle sticks, but a butter knife or the end of a spoon also works well.
- a clock, stopwatch or watch
- a bathroom scale and a tape measure

These tools are described in detail in "Your Home Health Center," page 208.

The Exam Itself

In this section, each part of the home physical exam is described:

how to do it, why, what you are looking for, and what to write down. On page 5 is a reduced figure of the Home Physical Exam form, found in "Family Medical Records," page 231.

VITAL SIGNS

Taking the vital signs is the easiest way to measure the life sustaining functions of the body. Vital signs can tell us much more than simply if a person is alive (vita means life in Greek). The 3 most essential vital signs are pulse (rate of heart beat), respiration (breath rate), and the body temperature. Monitoring your blood pressure, height, and weight is also valuable.

It is important to have records of a person's vital signs when the person is well to have a standard to compare against when the person falls ill.

Height and weight, besides being a record of a child's growth, can be useful in diagnosing an illness. Sudden weight loss or gain accompanies some illnesses. Weigh at the same time of day, undressed. Measure height without shoes.

Temperature, too, can be useful in diagnosis. Normal is 98.6° orally, but varies by individual, so it is important to determine a normal temperature for each person. Temperatures vary with time of day and other factors, so take the temperature 3 times a day, on several different days, to decide what is average.

In the *Healthwise Handbook,*

HOME PHYSICAL EXAM

Date _____ Name _____

Time of day _____

VITAL SIGNS

Height	Weight
Temperature Rectal Oral	Pulse Beats per minute? Regular?
Respiration Breaths per minute?	Blood Pressure

Reason for physical exam _____

Overall impression, comments _____

Mental health observations _____

Skin	Skull, hair, scalp
Eyes Pupil constriction:	Nose
Ears Hearing	Mouth, teeth

HOME PHYSICAL EXAM
(Continued)

Throat	Neck, lymph nodes Chin to chest:
Chest, breasts	Spine
Abdomen	Genitals
Anus Bowel movements	Legs and arms
Hands, nails	Feet, nails
Chest, lungs, heart sounds	Infants (under 2)
Adult women (over 18) Breast	

Additional comments: _____

Home physical exam forms

when reference to temperature is made, it will be an oral temperature. Since rectal and oral temperatures vary by only 1 degree, the difference is not critical, but you should know the kind of temperature if you need to discuss it with a health professional.

Details of how to take a temperature and measure the other vital signs are given at the end of this chapter, on page 19.

REASON FOR PHYSICAL

Write here why the exam is being done: person is ill, or routine check.

OVERALL IMPRESSIONS, COMMENTS

Include here a brief description of the person—attitude toward exam, general appearance, overall condition.

MENTAL HEALTH OBSERVATIONS

Note the child's general outlook (anxious, cheerful, depressed, etc.). Describe any self-stimulating behaviors such as thumbsucking, scratching, hair sucking, clinging to a favorite toy or blanket, or head banging. Regression to a behavior that has been given up earlier is of particular concern. Other behaviors or symptoms of mental health problems should be noted (see Chapter 11).

SKIN

Look at *all* the skin for overall tone and color. Look for moles, warts, bruises, cuts, boils, lumps, rashes, birthmarks, insect bites, etc. You're becoming familiar with the skin, so the next time you examine the person you can note any changes. The first time write down the size and location of everything you observe. In subsequent exams, note any changes. Record the condition of the skin: dry, oily, sweaty, etc.

SKULL, HAIR, SCALP

Learn what is normal. Feel the skull for lumps, bumps, or tender areas. Check the hair for cleanliness, shininess, bounce. When normally healthy hair looks dull, make a note to mention it at your next visit. Look for bald spots on the scalp, flakiness, or dandruff. Check for lice or other insects.

EYES

Check for crustiness or flaking on eyebrows or eyelashes. Look for matter in eyes, redness in whites of eyes, or excessive tearing. See page 68 for diagnosing these eye problems.

Pupil Constriction Test: Used to determine how a person's eyes ordinarily constrict, and after a head injury. In a darkened room, use a penlight. Direct the light from the right side into the right pupil. Watch the pupil constrict. Direct the light from the left side to the left pupil. Observe several times. Pupils should constrict to about the same size, at about the same rate. Some people normally have different-sized pupils. The importance is in establishing what is normal for each individual.

For a simple pupil constriction test when there is no injury, play "anybody home?". Instruct your child to cover eyes then put hands down. You look at pupils as soon as the hands are lowered.

NOSE

Check to see that the person breathes through both nostrils. Examine discharge, if any. Write down the color, and whether it is thick or thin. To better see the inside of the nose, flatten it and gently push up. Use a penlight to examine the tissues inside the nose. Note whether they are pink and healthy-looking or gray, blue, red, or inflamed. In a child, look for a sign of an object in the nose. If there is a foul odor from the nose, make a note of it. See Object in Nose, page 92, if any of these symptoms are found.

Apply firm pressure on the sinuses to test for tenderness.

EARS

Check the outer ear and behind the ear for crustiness, and wiggle the outer ear to test for tenderness. Use a penlight to look in the ear canal for wax. Pull the pinna (lobe) gently to see into the canal more clearly. Note if the wax is thin and runny, thick, brown, black, or whatever. Note, too, if there is a foul odor to the ear.

closer. Ask the person to tell you when the ticking is first heard. Repeat for the other ear. The sound should be heard at about the same distance away from each ear.

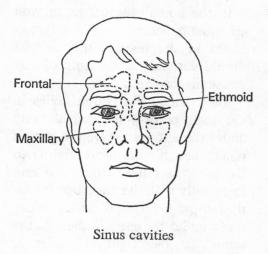

Sinus cavities

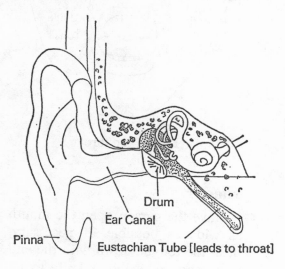

Ear

HEARING

The following simple test is a very rough check of hearing. Any possible problem discovered with this test should be thoroughly investigated by a health professional. The alert parent will also notice if a child suddenly doesn't respond to a simple question such as "Do you want to go to the movie?" Try not to use a question that may be normally ignored, such as "Ready for your bath?" or "Would you pick up your toys?".

Use a clock, watch, or some other object which makes a stable, quiet sound. Hold the clock out of sight some distance from one side of the person's head, and slowly move

MOUTH

Using a penlight, check inside the mouth for sores or white spots on the tongue, cheeks, or lips. Look at the teeth and gums. Healthy gums are pink, sometimes grayish, firm and strong. They grow tightly around each tooth. Record any tenderness, puffiness or bleeding in the gums or if the seal around the base of each tooth appears to be pulling away. Examine the teeth for black or brown spots or holes (possible cavities). Check to see if the teeth are clean or if there is obvious plaque. For a discussion of plaque, see page 164. Note new arrivals for children.

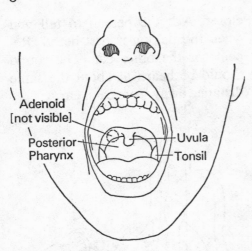

Adenoid
[not visible]

Posterior
Pharynx

Uvula

Tonsil

Mouth and throat

THROAT

Have the person open the mouth as wide as possible. If necessary, push the tongue down with the end of a spoon or a butter knife to let you see way back in the throat. Having a small child "pant like a puppy when he's hot" sometimes helps.

Using a penlight, check for swollen or bright red tonsils (if they are there). Healthy throat tissue is pink and moist. Note anything red, swollen, white or yellow. Notice if there is yellow or white mucus draining down the back of the throat (the pharynx).

NECK

Check the neck for swollen lymph nodes and for flexibility. The lymph system acts as a sort of filter for infection, destroying bacteria brought to the nodes by white blood cells. Lymph nodes are located throughout the body and will swell when there is an infection in a nearby part of the body. For example, the node at the groin would swell if there were an infected cut on the thigh.

In the home physical exam, you are most concerned with the lymph nodes in the neck, although you should certainly make note of any unusually swollen node.

To examine the lymph nodes in the neck, place your hand directly under the left jaw. Have the person relax, then tilt the head slightly to the left. Start under the chin and feel gently with the fingertips for little lumps, the lymph nodes. Work up to under the ear and then do the same for the right side. On a healthy adult, you won't feel the nodes. With a minor infection, the nodes may enlarge to the size of

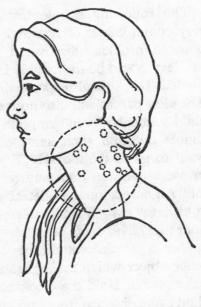

Lymph nodes of the neck

lima beans. However, children's lymph nodes may swell up enormously with an infection and not reduce for several weeks. History of past infections, and knowing what's normal for your child are important in this case.

The neck should also be examined for any unusual lumps or bumps. Cysts on the neck are fairly common in babies and young children. A cyst is an enclosed pouch or sac of skin, often filled with mucus or oil-like material. They are not serious, but should be reported to your health professional at the next visit.

Any enlarged lymph node or unusual lump for which you cannot find a reasonable cause should be reported to a health professional. Also check the neck for flexibility. Ask the person to touch chin to chest. If it cannot be done easily, this should be investigated.

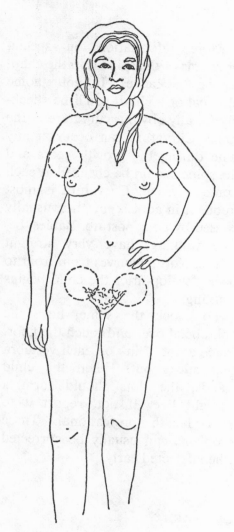

Lymph nodes of the body

CHEST, BREASTS

Newborns, male and female, often have some swelling in one or both breasts and sometimes there will be a secretion from the nipples. This is perfectly normal and it should go away in a few weeks. If not, see a health professional. Swelling of one or both breasts is also normal in some male adolescents, and is of no concern unless combined with redness, tenderness, or fever.

Look at the chest for symmetry (same on both sides) and to see how the person normally breathes —with chest or abdomen. Listen to breathing sounds—harshness, irregularity, raspiness, whistling, dry crackling, or gurgling sounds are signs to discuss with your health professional.

Women over 18 should examine their breasts monthly. See Self-breast Examination on page 16.

SPINE

More information on special problems of the spine is in the chapter on backaches. In your home physical of a child, you'll be checking for any obvious curvature of the spine. Curvature can occur at any time during the growth years and the spine should be checked at each home physical. Curvature is most frequent in adolescent girls, usually caused by poor posture. Babies, before walking, have very straight spines. Normal curves from front to back develop after the child begins walking.

To check the spine, have the child bend over and touch the floor. Place a dot of ink on each vertebra that sticks out. When the child stands, the dots should form a straight line. If not, report it to your health professional. These problems can usually be corrected when detected early.

ABDOMEN

Babies and young children normally have pot-bellies. As the child grows, the abdomen no longer sticks out.

To check the abdomen, divide it mentally into 4 areas or quadrants. The person should be undressed at least to the hair line of the pelvis. Make the person as comfortable as possible by putting a pillow under the head, and keeping the room comfortably warm. Have the person lie down, hands resting on chest, knees slightly bent.

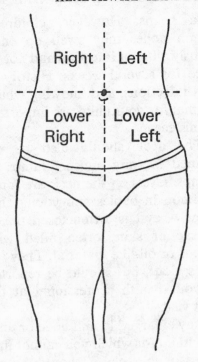

Abdominal quadrants

Notice whether the person's abdomen is normally flat or bulged out. In a young child you may find a bulging area at the navel. This is an umbilical hernia, which usually will go away in a few months. Sometimes they take 2–3 years to close up, but there is no cause for concern.

Feel the abdomen in all 4 quadrants, using hands as shown.

Press gently, asking if there is pain, and watching for flinching. Normally you will not be able to feel any organs. Note if you do feel any masses. Also make a note of any hard or rigid surfaces. A hard smooth mass at the center of the bottom of the abdomen is probably only a full bladder.

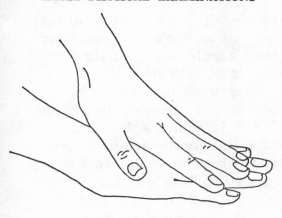

Hand position

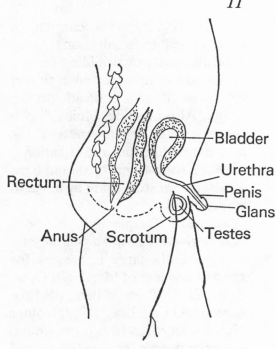

Rectum — Anus — Scrotum — Bladder — Urethra — Penis — Glans — Testes

Male genitals

Inguinal hernias are found in the groin, most frequently in males. To check for an inguinal hernia in males, look at the area just above the scrotum, at the groin, for any soft or bulging areas. This can be seen most easily if the person is coughing, laughing, or crying.

GENITALS

Male: In babies the size of the penis and scrotum will vary. Normally the testes are in the scrotum at birth or will descend in a short time. You and your health professional should watch for undescended testes. Occasional hardening (erection) of the penis is normal in babies and small boys. The decision to circumcise a boy is up to the parents and their health professional.

To examine a male's genitals, look at the penis for sores, red spots or "pimples." Now check the glans (the head of the penis covered by the foreskin) to see that the urinary opening (urethra) is at the tip of the glans. Sores are common in circumcised babies, so check carefully. In uncircumcised babies, do not force the foreskin back. A waxy substance is a normal lubricant.

Check also the scrotum, the sac which holds the testes. Note any sores or red areas. Notice in a baby whether the testes have come down into the scrotum. Gently squeeze. You should feel 2, 1 in each side of the scrotum, about the size of a kidney bean. The testes and scrotum enlarge when a boy is about 10 to 13 years old.

There should be no pain or discomfort on urination. Urine should come out in a fairly steady stream, without straining. Urine should be pale yellow and there should not be a strong ammonia odor, which is a sign the urine is too concentrated (a clue to possible dehydration).

Strain, pain, or dribbling on urination are symptoms which should be discussed with a health professional. Also swelling, bluish discoloration, pain, or tenderness of the scrotum require medical attention.

Males over 40 or 45 should have an annual prostate exam by a health professional.

Female: Frequently, newborn baby girls have swollen genitals and a vaginal discharge is present for the first 2 weeks of life. A girl's genitals include 2 sets of lips called the inner (labia minora) and the outer (labia majora), which form around the urinary opening and the vaginal opening. In babies the inside lips and the clitoris (the front part where the 2 lips come together) stick out much more than when the girl is older. The outside lips look like a red cuff around the vaginal opening. The redness fades as the baby grows. The lips are sometimes stuck together but generally separate as the baby grows.

Later sexual development in girls usually begins between the ages of 9 and 11 with a widening of the hips, hair growing under the arms and in the pubic area, and enlarging of the breasts. These changes usually take place before menstruation begins.

Examine the entire genital area for any sores, red swollen areas, or discharge. The area inside the 2 lips should be pink and moist.

There should be no pain or straining on urination and the urine should come out in a fairly steady stream. The color should be pale yellow and there should be no strong ammonia odor.

Most women should have a yearly Pap smear test to detect early stages of cancer of the cervix.

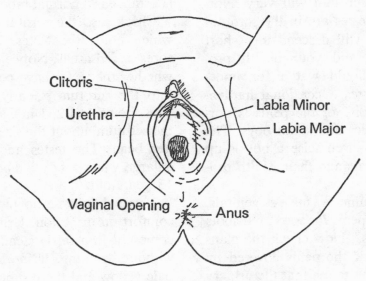

Female genitals

Cancer detected at this early stage is almost always curable. Do not douche on the day of your Pap smear or make an appointment during your menstrual period. Also don't go when you have a vaginal infection; treat it first. All of these conditions can make the test inaccurate.

Normally a mature woman should start having exams when sexual activity begins. There appears to be a connection between level of sexual activity, especially with multiple partners, and cancer of the cervix. Therefore, a 16-year-old who is having sexual relations should have an exam at 16. After the first exam, women should have yearly exams.

ANUS

The anus is the opening where the bowel movement or stool comes out. This area is usually darker in color than the surrounding skin and is wrinkled together when closed. It stretches to let a bowel movement out and then closes again.

Check for cuts or sores beside the anus, and for swelling. Bright red blood in the stools probably indicates there are fissures (little splits or tears) in the skin of the anus. These should be seen by a health professional.

A black or tarry stool can be a sign of internal bleeding and should be brought to the immediate attention of your health professional.

You should know what the regular pattern of bowel movements is for each family member. Make a note of it on the exam record. Remember that "regular" does not mean daily. See Constipation, page 29.

LEGS AND ARMS

The legs and arms should each be of equal length. Check to see if one shoulder blade is higher than the other. Many people have one limb slightly shorter than the other, but it is important to know what is normal for each person.

Look for swollen joints, especially the ankles. Move the arms and legs in a full range of motion to test for flexibility. Record any stiffness or pain on movement.

For walking children, check to see that the child walks normally, with no shuffling, staggering, or discomfort. A 3-year-old often has knock-knees, but usually outgrows these in a couple of years.

HANDS AND NAILS

Examine the hands for calluses, warts, and sores. See whether both hands are about the same size and opposing fingers the same length. Nails should be clean and trimmed and not brittle or peeling.

Newborn babies have very strong grips. This is a reflex which disappears as a baby develops. You should check for a good firm grip in everyone. Also become familiar with the size and shape of fingers so any later thickening or clubbing will be recognized.

FEET AND NAILS

Check the feet for sore spots or calluses, for unusual lumps, and for plantar's warts on the sole of the foot. See Warts, page 123. Both feet should be similar in length and toes, too, should match. When the person is standing, there should be some open space between the ball of the foot and heel—the arch. However, little babies all have "flat feet." It is a fat pad that disappears with growth. Usually even quite "flat" feet aren't a problem unless the person has discomfort when walking. Look between the toes for any sign of infection such as athlete's foot. Check the nails for brittleness, peeling, or infection.

Move the legs and feet about to check for flexibility or pain on movement.

LUNG AND HEART SOUNDS

This exam is only useful if you have a stethoscope. Place ear pieces of the stethoscope into the ears, pointing forward, toward the eardrum. Place the stethoscope on the person's back. Listen all over the back above the waistline to the right and left of the spine. You are listening to learn what normal breathing sounds are for that person, so you can recognize when there is a change from normal. Ask the person to take a deep breath through the mouth and exhale slowly.

Repeat this process, with the stethoscope on the chest. If the person is a hairy-chested male, you will hear the hairs scratch against the stethoscope. With a fleshy or heavily-muscled person you may not be able to hear any breath sounds.

Next listen for the heartbeat. Place the stethoscope near the nipple about 3 inches left of the middle of the chest. You will hear a lub-dub sound. Count the heartbeats, which are the same as the pulse. On a weakened or severely ill person this may be the only way to get a heart rate. If you notice a sound other than normal, it may be a possible heart murmur and should be recorded and reported to a health professional at your next visit. A heart murmur has a sssh! sound, but is really rather difficult for the lay person to recognize. Learn to distinguish normal from abnormal.

Facts About Infants

The following brief notes are of particular concern to parents of infants (birth to 1 year). They may dispel some unnecessary parental fears.

The umbilical cord will drop off and the navel will usually heal in 1–3 weeks. At the time the cord comes off, there may be a moist or bloody oozing for a few days. This does not need special treatment. After leaving the hospital, clean the navel daily with a bit of cotton wet with rubbing alcohol. Discontinue this when the navel is healed. Do not give a pan or tub bath until the navel is healed. The appearance of the navel is not affected by the way the cord is tied off. Bellybands will not prevent an umbilical hernia (bulging out). Hernias usually go away within a year, although sometimes it will take several years.

Newborns frequently have rashes or white "pimples" scattered over their bodies which usually clear without treatment. Often the skin will peel or flake off during the first 2–3 weeks after birth. This is normal and requires no treatment.

Many babies have no tear ducts for the first few months of life. In some babies, tears will spill out. These tears are not problems and need no treatment.

Ears on newborns may be soft and floppy. The cartilage has not yet hardened but it will become firm as the baby grows.

Often there is hair on the face or body of a newborn. This will go away in a few months. The head may be misshapen but will round out in a few days.

An infant may commonly snort and sneeze during the first few weeks of life. This rarely indicates a cold. Hiccups and spitting are also common.

Bowel movements resemble tar the first day or so.

You should check infants for hip dislocation (the hip bone is not in its socket):

1. Check the thigh folds. If the hip is dislocated, one thigh fold will be higher than the other.
2. When the child is lying face up with thighs and knees bent, as in Position 1, legs should be the same length. If one leg appears shorter than the other, there is a possibility of hip dislocation.
3. In the same position, when legs are bent outward as in Position 2, legs should bend outward to the same distance.

Any abnormalities should be reported to a health professional. When discovered early, hip dislocation is easily corrected. Late correction is difficult and time-consuming.

Checking for hip dislocation

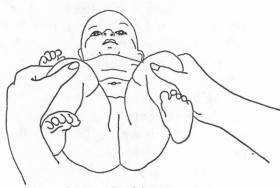

Position 1

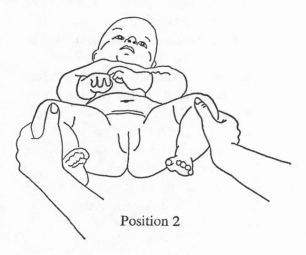

Position 2

Self-breast Examination

Of special concern to adult women is the breast examination. Women over age 18 should start a monthly habit of examining their breasts.

Breast cancer is the number one cancer killer among women, yet, if caught early, it is highly curable. Over 95% of breast lumps are discovered by women themselves, so it is very important for each woman to take responsibility for checking her breasts monthly.

Establish a regular time each month to examine your breasts. A good time is a few days after your menstrual period, for the breasts will not be swollen or tender. Menopausal women can examine their breasts the first day of each month. After hysterectomy, check with your health professional for an appropriate time.

Begin your breast examination in the shower or bath when your hands are wet and soapy and glide easily over the skin. With your fingers flat, move gently over every part of each breast. Use your left hand to examine the right breast. Check for lumps or thickening.

Next examine your breasts visually before a mirror. You are looking for any dimpling, puckering, retraction of the skin, or any changes in the contour of the breast. A monthly examination will help you become familiar with your body so you can recognize any changes. Next, lift the arms above the head and again inspect the breasts.

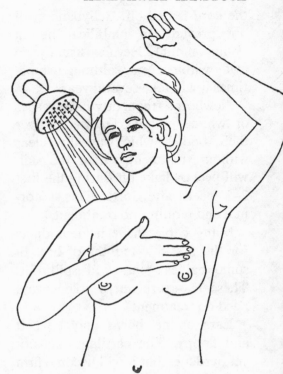

Self-breast examination—starts in the shower

Few women have left and right breasts that match exactly. Learn what is normal for you.

Now place the heels of your hands together in front of your chest and press together. Again, look for dimpling or any skin changes.

The third step of the breast examination is done lying down. Place a pillow or a folded towel under the shoulder of the side you will examine. Place your arm at your side. Use your right hand to examine the left breast. With fingers relaxed, use the flats of the fingers in gentle circular motions, and examine the inside of the breast. Be

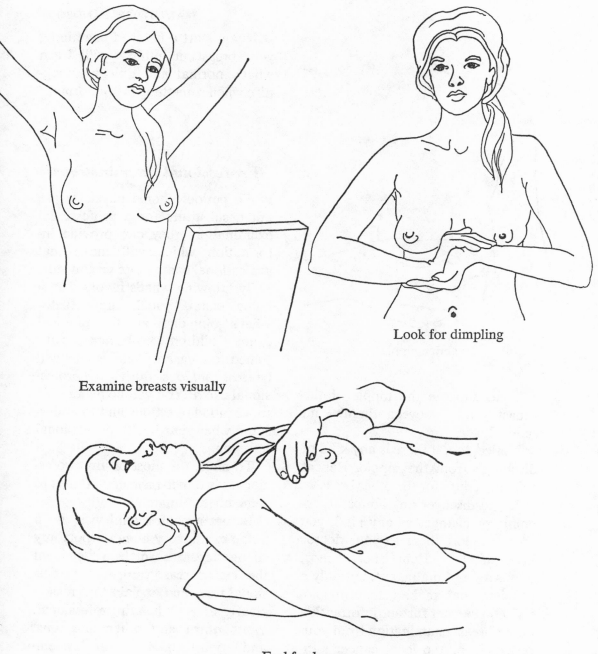

Examine breasts visually

Look for dimpling

Feel for lumps

sure to cover all the breast tissue, with particular attention to the nipple area. Feel the area over the breastbone (sternum) also.

You are feeling for lumps, thickening, or changes of any kind. To examine the outside of the breast, place your left arm under your head. Now using the flat of your fingers, in a circular motion, examine all the tissue on the outside of the breast. Feel up under the arm and high into the armpit for possible lumps.

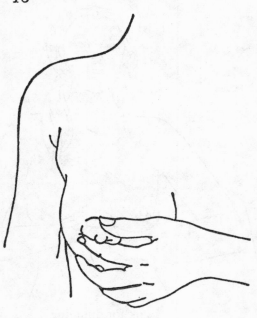

Examine nipples

If you start a habit of examining your breasts monthly, you'll learn what's normal and quickly recognize when something is not normal.

Professional Examinations

While periodic home physicals are not a substitute for a professional examination, they can provide information which will make that professional exam more worthwhile.

By knowing what's involved in a home exam, you'll know better what's going on in an office physical exam. Children who become accustomed to pleasant home exams will be less anxious during a professional exam. You will be better able to ask good questions and to understand what your health professional tells you.

To make the most of any professional visit, there are a few things to remember.

Before a professional visit, do a home exam, so you can report any changes from normal. Write down the major reason for the professional visit, and explain that reason clearly to your health professional. Write down any other questions, and go through them systematically. If you do not understand what your health professional is saying, ask questions. Get clear answers to your questions before you leave the office.

If an illness is diagnosed, ask what, if anything, you can do to

Next, squeeze the nipple of the breast gently between thumb and index finger.

Notice, too, if there is any kind of discharge from the nipple. Repeat this procedure for the other breast.

If you discover any lumps, thickening, or changes of any kind, you should report these to your doctor immediately. Remember, most lumps are not malignant, but only a physician can make a final diagnosis. You can get further information about breast examination from your physician or the local cancer society.

If you detect cysts in your breast, draw a diagram of your breast and mark the location of the cysts. You will easily find them the next month to determine if they have changed or you have others.

speed recovery. Is bed rest necessary? Will steam help? Many things besides a shot or a prescription can aid a cure. If a prescription is given, be sure you understand how to use the drug. Also ask about possible side effects, and what to do if they occur. Ask if there may be a less expensive, but comparable substitute.

Be sure you understand all recommended treatments and why they should help. Also, if something sounds impossible, tell the health professional. "There's no way I can stay in bed all day with 3 kids!" Together you can work out a suitable solution.

Ask about restrictions on activity and how long the restriction is necessary.

Try to get a picture of what to expect. "Jennie should feel better in 2 days, but keep her in bed for 3 full days and on the medication for 10 days." After the visit, call if something unexpected happens.

If you are concerned about the accuracy of a diagnosis, talk it over with your health professional or ask for a second opinion or consultation. Most physicians will agree readily.

If the visit is for a child's examination you may wish to take with you:

1. immunization records
2. a urine sample in a clean container
3. any abnormal stool or vomit (if that is the reason for the visit)

Measuring Vital Signs

HOW TO TAKE A TEMPERATURE

A fever is body temperature that is raised abnormally. An active person on a hot day may have a temperature of 100° Fahrenheit (F.) without being ill at all.

If there is a normal reason for a slightly higher temperature and the person otherwise seems okay, there is no cause for concern.

Normal temperature can range from 97.6 to 99.6° orally. Fever occurs when the body is trying to fight off an infection. A higher body temperature helps the body fight off infection, but too high a fever can be harmful. There is no medical need to reduce a temperature until it is over 102° orally, but you may wish to reduce the fever if the person is uncomfortable.

The person with a fever needs to drink extra water, as fever burns off body liquids faster.

Temperatures can be taken 3 ways:

1. orally, in the mouth under the tongue
2. axillary, in the armpit
3. rectally, in the anus

Generally, a rectal temperature is good for small children but requires careful attention. An axillary temperature avoids the danger of the thermometer breaking in the mouth or anus but is not as accurate. Use it only when other methods are not possible. An oral temperature is simplest for adults and older children.

Although the thermometers can be used interchangeably, a rectal thermometer is fatter and thicker, so it breaks less easily.

An oral temperature is ordinarily about 1 degree higher than an axillary temperature and 1 degree lower than a rectal temperature. That is, if the rectal temperature is 101°, the oral would be 100° and the axillary (armpit) 99°.

Indicate the method you use when you report the temperature to your health professional. "The temperature is 99.8° orally." In this handbook, temperatures will always be given as oral temperatures.

Procedure:

- Wash off the bulb, where the mercury is, and the lower part of the thermometer with cool, soapy water or rubbing alcohol. Hold the thermometer tightly by the end opposite the bulb and "shake it down," as if you were trying to shake drops of water off the bulb. This is needed to lower the mercury below 95° on the thermometer. Since the thermometer can easily slip from your hand, shake it over a bed or soft object.
- In taking the oral temperature, be sure the lips are closed. Have the person breathe through the nose. This may be more difficult with a stuffy nose. In tak-

ing the axillary temperature, press the arm close to the body for 5 minutes. For rectal and oral temperatures, keep the thermometer in place for 3 minutes.

- A good way to take a rectal temperature is to place the infant or child on your lap, bottom up. Hold the child still with one hand and insert the thermometer with the other.
- To read a thermometer: note that the thermometer

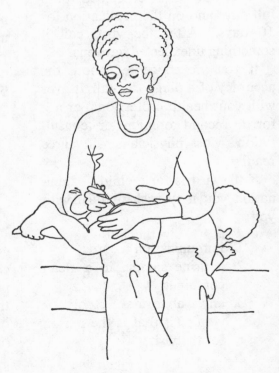

Taking a rectal temperature

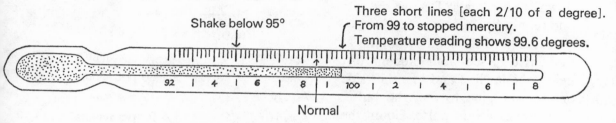

Shake below 95°

Three short lines [each 2/10 of a degree].
From 99 to stopped mercury.
Temperature reading shows 99.6 degrees.

92 | 4 | 6 | 8 | 100 | 2 | 4 | 6 | 8

Normal

Reading a thermometer

is graduated from 92 degrees to 108 degrees. Each large mark indicates 1 degree of temperature. Between large marks are 5 small marks. Each small mark stands for 0.2 degrees (2/10).

- Read the thermometer in good light. Holding the end opposite the mercury bulb, rotate the thermometer slowly until you can see a silver (sometimes red) ribbon of mercury. The place where this ribbon stops indicates the temperature reading. Write it down, noting the kind of temperature (oral, rectal, axillary), and the time of day.

HOW TO MEASURE PULSE RATE

Measuring the pulse rate is one simple way to count a person's heartbeats. Contractions of the heart muscles as they force blood throughout the body cause a throbbing in the arteries. The pulse is actually the heartbeat.

A pulse can be taken wherever an artery comes close to the skin sur-

face. Usually it is taken at the wrist, but often it's easier at the neck.

The pulse should be counted after the person has been resting quietly, or for a child, while asleep.

To take the pulse at the wrist, place 2 fingers against the wrist as shown (not the thumb, you may feel *your* pulse). Have the person raise the thumb to make a natural pocket for your fingers. Count the beats for 30 seconds then double the results. The pulse is measured by beats per minute. After you count the pulse, keep your fingers on the artery and feel for regularity —does the pulse speed up or slow

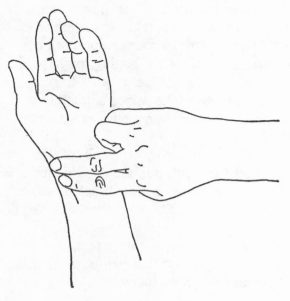

Taking a pulse rate

down or skip beats? Record the rate and regularity.

If it is hard to feel a throbbing at the wrist, place your fingers just below the jawline and to either side of the windpipe to feel the pulse. This is the carotid pulse. Count the beats for 30 seconds and double the results. The pulse rate is the same no matter where you feel it.

Pulse rate rises about 10 beats with each degree of fever.

Normal Resting Pulse Rates

Adults	60–100 beats per minute
6–10 years	70–110 beats per minute
Infant–1 year	70–150 beats per minute

HOW TO MEASURE RESPIRATION

Respiration rate is how many breaths a person takes in a minute. The best time to count respiration is when the person is resting, perhaps after taking the pulse with fingers still at pulse. The person's breathing is apt to change on seeing you count it.

Count the rise and fall of the chest for 1 full minute. Also notice whether there is any "sucking-in" beneath the ribs or other abnormality.

Record the respiration rate.

As a person's temperature rises, respiration rates increase.

Normal Resting Respiration Rates

Newborn	30–80 per minute
One Year	20–40 per minute
Age 6	12–19 per minute
Age 10	17–22 per minute
Adult	15–20 per minute

HOW TO TAKE A BLOOD PRESSURE

If you have a blood pressure cuff (sphygmomanometer) and a stethoscope.

Blood pressure is the force of the flowing blood against the walls of the arteries. *Systolic* pressure is the pressure when the heart contracts and pumps the blood through the body. *Diastolic* pressure is pressure between pumps, when the heart is relaxing.

Most blood pressure cuffs are for adults and are too large for a child's small arm. When it is necessary to measure a child's blood pressure, your health professional has a child-sized cuff.

Procedure:

- Have the person seated beside a table, with a bare arm outstretched. Loosen the valve by turning it counterclockwise and deflate the cuff completely.
- Wrap the blood pressure cuff snugly around the person's arm with the lower edge of the cuff 1 inch

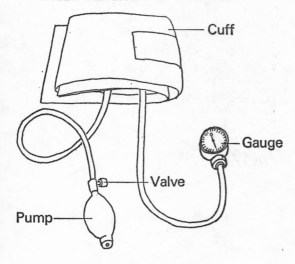

Blood pressure cuff

above the crease at the elbow. Be sure the tubing going to the bulb is closest to the patient's body and the tubing going to the gauge is away from the body.

• Feel for the person's pulse in the bend of the elbow. Place the stethoscope there.

• Close the valve of the bulb and pump the bulb to raise pressure to a level of about 160 on the gauge. If you hear a heartbeat right away, then pump it up higher. Immediately loosen the valve a bit so the needle starts moving down slowly. Don't leave the cuff pumped up; the pressure hurts.

• Watch the dial as you listen with the stethoscope. You will soon hear a tapping sound—the pulse sounds. The number on the dial when you first hear the pulse sounds is the systolic pressure. A typical systolic pressure might be 125.

• As air continues to escape from the cuff, the sounds will eventually disappear completely. Note where the needle is when the sounds disappear. This is the diastolic pressure. A normal example would be 70.

• Open the valve completely, let the pressure fall to zero, and remove the cuff.

• Record the reading, systolic/diastolic (125/70 for above example).

If you need to recheck your measurement, be sure the cuff is entirely deflated before inflating it again. Otherwise, your new measurement will be inaccurate. If you cannot get a clear reading after 2 tries, use the other arm, or wait 5 full minutes.

An adult under age 60 has a normal blood pressure of under 140/90. Anything over that should be reported to a health professional.

Taking a blood pressure reading correctly requires practice. You should review the procedure with your health professional.

2

Abdominal Problems

Sooner or later some form of stomach pain affects us all. Although most such abdominal problems are minor and require only our casual attention, other stomachaches can be caused by serious, life-threatening conditions. Between the green-apple stomachache and the trauma of acute appendicitis lie a number of common stomach problems for which appropriate home care can best speed recovery.

Abdominal pain usually results from some disorder in the digestive system. When the stomach and intestines are irritated by infections, food poisons, ulcers, or obstructions, their functions of digestion, water absorption, and waste removal are disrupted.

By closely observing these changes and by examining general symptoms such as pain, temperature, and vital signs, a person can better understand and deal with abdominal problems.

Whenever you are worried about an abdominal pain, first go through the home physical exam discussed on page 3. Remember, it is the whole person you are worried about, not just the person's stomach. The exam may uncover some important information about the problem. Next focus on the abdominal area. Use the abdominal pain history and exam questions on page 26, to find out as much as you can about the problem. Be sure to write down anything that may be helpful later in describing the problem to a health professional.

Of course, if your patient is a very small child, or a very old person, you may not be able to get good answers to many of the questions. In such cases added caution is always advised.

In most cases, parents who know their children and are aware of the most likely causes of bellyache will be able to figure out what's going on. *Remember though, the cause of abdominal pain is sometimes very*

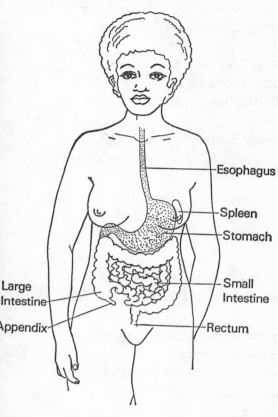

Digestive tract

- Esophagus
- Spleen
- Stomach
- Small Intestine
- Rectum
- Large Intestine
- Appendix

available should the conditions worsen.

Many of the common causes of abdominal pain and other stomach problems are discussed throughout this section. The information provided, together with some common sense and the answers to the history question on page 26 should give you a good basis for safely handling a stomachache at home or for effectively relating the problem to a health professional.

Appendicitis

The appendix is a small, apparently useless, sac extending from the large bowel. The digestive fluids circulate through it and cleanse it of any bacteria. However, if its normal opening becomes plugged, the bacteria can build up and cause a serious infection, appendicitis.

Sometimes the opening is plugged by objects passing through the intestines—pebbles, seeds, toothpicks, small bones, and clumps of hair. More often, the appendix becomes blocked by its own twisting or by small hard bits of bowel material.

The real danger is in the appendix bursting. That spreads the infection to other vital organs which can cause serious problems. Fortunately, that isn't going to happen 5 minutes after your first pain. Usually the pain builds up for 12 hours or more before an appendix bursts. Some people have very high tolerance to pain, however, and may not

serious and difficult for even a health professional to diagnose. Any time abdominal pain is either severe or persistent, or increasing over several hours, a health professional should be called. Cramps due to gas can be very painful. However, a doctor doesn't need to be seen unless the cramps are not diminished by the passage of gas, stools, or several hours of restful observation. *If any doubt exists regarding the cause or severity of the pain, a phone call to your health professional is strongly recommended.* He or she can then evaluate your observations and be readily

Abdominal Pain: History and Exam

- When did the pain first appear?
    Has it been constant, increasing, off and on?
    What is the location of the pain? Has the location changed?
    What is the "quality" of the pain? (Sharp, burning, dull.)
    Is it painful to urinate?
- Is the patient's skin clammy or does the patient appear to be in shock?
- What are the patient's temperature and pulse as compared to their normal rates? (Retake every few hours.)
- Does the abdomen appear unusual in size, shape or rigidity? Is it tender to the touch?
- Is there any blood or unusual color in the urine?
- Is the patient's saliva sticky? Slippery?
- Has the patient vomited? Or been nauseated? How much? How often?
- Has the patient had recent contact with anyone else with similar pain? Or similar symptoms?
- Has the patient consumed an unusual amount or type of food or drink?
- Has the patient eaten any unrefrigerated meats recently?
- Has the patient sustained any recent sharp blow or injury to the stomach?
- Has the patient been under unusually heavy stress lately?
- Has the patient appeared nervous or tense?

---

notice it for several hours after it begins.

Appendicitis is not common in very young children. However, since small children cannot describe their pain well, their cases often become quite serious before they are diagnosed.

HOME TREATMENT

- Perform basics of home physical exam including vital signs. See home physical exam, page 3.
- Watch for and record any of the following symptoms:
    o Abdominal pain preceded by period of nausea and loss of appetite. Although the pain may first be very general or seem to come from any point in the abdomen, it will usually move to the right lower quadrant as it increases.
    o Vomiting or increasing nausea.
    o Low grade fever of 100–101°.
    o Notice any bowel movements. Diarrhea is rarely present with appendicitis and can be a good clue that the pain

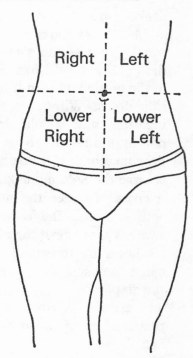

Abdominal quadrants

is due to some other cause. Good bowel movements are very common with appendicitis.

- Keep the patient quiet and in a comfortable position.
- Try to identify or rule out other sources of abdominal pain such as food poisoning, gastroenteritis, or overeating.
- *DO NOT* give laxatives. They can stimulate the intestine and cause the appendix to rupture sooner.
- *DO NOT* give strong pain medication. Since the location and intensity of pain are diagnostic clues, the heavy use of aspirin or stronger pain reducers may hide important information.
- *DO NOT* apply heat to the area.

WHEN TO CALL A HEALTH PROFESSIONAL

- If any of the above symptoms cause you to suspect appendicitis you should call your health professional. The call is a must if the pain is in the lower right quadrant or is increasing steadily. The call will alert your health professional to the possible problem should assistance become necessary.

Colic

Colic is a problem of which the parents of young babies are often painfully aware. Colic is not really a disease. Rather it is a name we give to a whole assortment of problems that can cause babies to draw up their legs, tighten their abdomens and holler. First determine if the child is hungry. If the baby has just eaten and is still upset, it's a good chance colic is the problem.

Colic may often be caused because the child's digestive tract has not completely developed for handling milk. Also, any abnormality in feeding may bring on the problem. The most common include:

- Swallowing air because of feeding too fast, too slow or while lying down.
- Taking overheated milk.
- Using nipple holes that are too small.
- Nervous tension in the family during feeding.
- Intolerance to sugar in the formula.
- Allergy to cow's milk.

The same symptoms could also be caused by a tight rectal muscle or by pain elsewhere in the body (earache, hernia, or urinary infection).

The nice thing about colic is that it goes away as the baby's system matures, almost always by the end of the third month. Of course, it's over sooner for many babies and may never appear in many others. Although no one method always works to relieve colicky babies, there are a number of possible remedies you can try.

HOME TREATMENT

- Most important—stay calm and try to relax.
- Make sure the child is getting enough to eat—the problem may be hunger, not colic.
- Prop the baby up during and for 15 minutes after feeding. "Burp" the baby after each ounce.
- Don't overheat the formula but heat to body temperature.

- Make sure manufactured nipple holes aren't too small. To test the size of the hole, put cold formula in the bottle and turn it upside down. Without shaking, the milk should drip out at a rate of about 1 drop a second. If it doesn't, enlarge the hole by making a cross cut over the hole with a knife. Babies can swallow more air if the nipple holes are too small because they suck air around the nipple.
- Try a different cow's milk preparation, or use a milk substitute.
- Use a pacifier, and try rocking or walking the baby. Putting the baby stomach-down over your knee may be helpful.
- Don't worry about spoiling a baby the first 3 months; comforting babies makes them and you feel better.
- Get a friend or neighbor to baby-sit some evening while you go to dinner and a movie!
- If nothing else works, colic medicines are available to help relax the baby's stomach and intestinal muscles. They require a prescription. Be sure to ask your pharmacist to explain the correct dosage and any possible side effects the drug might cause.

- Don't feel guilty about shutting the bedroom door and turning up the stereo once in a while—if it will help you to relax, it will help the baby.

WHEN TO CALL A HEALTH PROFESSIONAL

- Colic normally does not require professional treatment unless it is accompanied by vomiting and/or diarrhea or other signs of more serious illness. If the child looks healthy between episodes and if your emotions can stand the noise for the first 3 months, you have little cause for worry.

Constipation

Constipation is the passage of hard, dry stools. If you pass soft stools, you are not constipated regardless of how "regularly" or "irregularly" you may pass them. The need for a bowel movement every day is a misconception. Some people pass stools every 3–5 days. As long as the stools are soft, such frequencies do not indicate constipation.

One of the chief causes of constipation is lack of time. The person who has had trouble with constipation should set aside a time each day, or as frequently as is normally needed, to go to the bathroom. Your bowels send you signals when there is a need to pass a movement. However, if you don't take time to heed the signal, after a while the urge will pass. Since the large intestine draws water from the stools, the stools will eventually become dry and difficult to pass. This postponing the inevitable is an all too frequent occurrence with children. Parents should be aware of their children's bowel habits, but try to relax and not make a big fuss about them. Stress can cause or add to a constipation problem. In children, stress related to toilet training may contribute to constipation problems.

PREVENTION

Diet is very important in constipation. Too much cow's milk for infants and too few fruits, juices and clear liquids can create the problem. Pregnant women are especially susceptible to constipation and should pay close attention to the amount of liquids in their diets. Susceptible people should increase the fiber in their diets by eating more bran cereals, apples, and celery. Regular exercise may also help prevent constipation.

HOME TREATMENT

Ages 0–1:

- Add water to formula or reduce breast feeding and add water.
- One teaspoon to 2 ounces of juice per feeding.

- Strained prunes: ½ to 3 tablespoons daily.
- If constipation persists after 3 days of the above treatment, do home physical exam to look for other possible problems.

Ages 2–12:

- Arrange for regular, relaxed time for bowel movements.
- Add fruits, vegetables, and liquids.
- Add lots of water—especially in the morning.
- Avoid laxatives if possible. Very few children need them and they can cause a laxative habit if overused. See Laxatives, page 226. *Never* use a laxative if abdominal pain is present. See Appendicitis, page 25.
- If a very acute episode occurs with hard painful stools, a mild stool softener or laxative may be used—but very sparingly. Ask your pharmacist to suggest one or review the examples on page 226.
- Discuss with the child any fears or stress related to toilet training or the passage of stools.

Adults:

- Set aside relaxed times for bowel movements.
- Add juice and fruits.
- Drink 2–4 extra glasses of water per day, especially in the morning.
- Avoid laxatives if possible. If necessary, use a stool softener or very mild laxative. Do not use mineral oil or any other laxative regularly. Mineral oil slows the body's absorption of vitamins. See Laxatives, page 226.

WHEN TO CALL A HEALTH PROFESSIONAL

- If constipation persists after the above treatment is followed for 3 days for babies or 1 week for adults.
- If dark blood is seen in stools. Small amounts of bright blood are usually caused by slight tearing as the stool is pushed through the anus and should stop when the constipation is controlled. More than a few streaks of bright blood should be discussed with a health professional.
- If constipation and major changes in bowel movement patterns occur and persist without apparent reason.

Dehydration

Dehydration is the excessive loss of water from the body. A continuous supply of water is required by all living cells in your body. When you stop consuming water or when you lose large amounts of fluids through diarrhea or sweat, body cells reabsorb fluid from the blood and other stores of water. If dehydration is allowed to continue, so much of the blood's fluids can be reabsorbed that the blood vessels collapse in vascular shock. Death then follows very quickly.

Because dehydration is extremely dangerous for infants and small children, it is important to watch closely for its early signs if vomiting, diarrhea, or both threaten to limit fluid intake. Fortunately, there are several good ways to test for dehydration. If you tried these tests when your child was normal, you will be better able to judge the test results.

DEHYDRATION TEST

- Feel the child's saliva. If it's wet and slippery, that's good. If it becomes dry and sticky, it could be an early sign of dehydration.
- A second test for the observant parent is to watch how much urine the child passes. A dehydrated baby will have darker, more concentrated urine and a diaper that is much less wet than normal.
- Look at the child. As dehydration progresses to more critical stages, the child's overall appearance will change. A dehydrated

child will look sick and have "sunken eyes."
- If when you pinch the skin on a child's tummy it feels doughy and doesn't snap right back, dehydration may have progressed to a very serious level.
- A dehydrated child's pulse rate will be faster than normal.

HOME TREATMENT

Treatment of mild dehydration is simple. First, stop the fluid loss. Then, restore lost fluids as soon as possible.

- If the child is nauseated or vomiting, stop all food and liquids for 2–4 hours to rest the stomach.
- As soon as vomiting is controlled, give clear liquids a little at a time until the stomach will accept larger amounts. You may start by giving the child 1 teaspoon of liquid every 10 minutes for 1–2 hours before increasing the amount. Don't give too much at one time.
- Do not give aspirin unless the fever is over 102°—it may further irritate the stomach. Tylenol or other aspirin substitutes may be less irritating.
- A potassium salt electrolyte solution or a drink like Gatorade may be advantageously substituted for

water since it will restore some of the salts lost with the fluids. See page 221 for how to make the solution.

- Continue to check the signs of dehydration for improvement or changes for the worse.

Since lots of fluids are needed to speed recovery from most minor illnesses, even mild dehydration can extend the length and severity of common health problems. Dehydration prevention and treatment should be considered *any time anyone* becomes ill.

WHEN TO CALL A HEALTH PROFESSIONAL

- If the child cannot hold down the small amounts of liquid given.
- If sick, sunken eye appearance develops.
- If there has been little or no urine for 12 hours.
- If the skin is doughy.
- If you cannot stop the fluid loss, the child may have to be hospitalized and given fluids intravenously.
- If temperature of 102° develops.

Diarrhea

Diarrhea is the discharge of watery stools, usually repeated several times a day. The presence of mildly loose stools at regular bowel movement times is not usually considered diarrhea and is not a cause of great concern.

Diarrhea is caused when the intestines become over-stimulated to empty themselves and push the stools through before the water in them can be reabsorbed by the body. Usually the stimulation is caused by some infection or irritation in the digestive tract. Since the body can best heal the infection if the intestine is empty, the initial effect of diarrhea can aid healing.

Diarrhea is a frequent occurrence for infants and small children. An infant's still-developing digestive system will sometimes not tolerate excessive amounts of fruit, juice or even milk. Although food tolerance diarrhea is upsetting and certainly messy, it usually presents no cause for concern. As long as the child appears healthy and is growing normally, no real treatment of occasional diarrhea is required. However, when the diarrhea becomes excessive, the problem foods must be found and temporarily eliminated from the diet. Of course, food allergies are not the only cause of diarrhea in infants. Organic disease such as gastroenteritis or GI flu must also be suspected.

Because of a child's small size and high need for fluids, excessive diarrhea can quickly dehydrate an infant's body. Although untreated dehydration can be very serious, careful observation of the child's appearance and fluid intake can prevent possible complications. See discussion on dehydration, page 30.

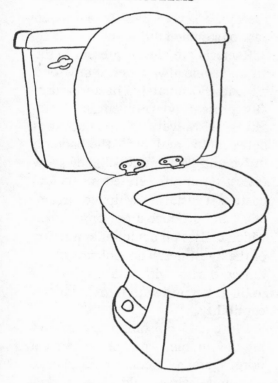

Diarrhea in adults is often brought on by nervousness, tension or emotional problems. It's your body's way of getting you to calm down. See page 200 for a discussion on how to cope with stress.

Acute diarrhea is often accompanied by abdominal discomfort and periodic cramping pain that is relieved by passing diarrhea. Should other pain develop or the discomfort increase, it may signal a more serious abdominal problem. In such a case a call to your physician is advised. The professional experience can help you decide if a visit is needed.

Chronic or intermittent diarrhea lasting over weeks or months may be caused by one of many life-threatening conditions which require professional help and labora-

tory tests to identify. Prolonged diarrhea also leads to a secondary problem of malnutrition and fluid loss since nutrients are passed before the body can absorb them.

HOME TREATMENT

- PUT YOUR STOMACH AT REST.
- Clear liquids only for the first 24 hours. (A clear liquid is one you can see through—milk is not clear.)
- Bed rest if possible— reduce activities.
- Mild foods can be added the next day.
- Spicy foods, fruit, alcohol, and coffee should be avoided until 48 hours after all symptoms have disappeared.
- Since diarrhea may sometimes speed recovery, anti-diarrheal drugs should be avoided for the first 6 hours and then used only if cramping or discomfort continues. See discussion on anti-diarrheal drugs, page 220.
- For small babies, temporarily substitute water for milk or formula in the diet. (An ounce of water at a time until the stomach has settled.) After several feedings, milk or diluted formula may be reintroduced. Breast milk feeding should be reduced too.

- A nursing mother may have to express her milk for a time.

- If the diarrhea is tarry or bloody. If the blood is bright red and there isn't much, it probably is only a scratch or fissure in the rectal area.
- If the diarrhea does not improve after 24 hours of clear liquids only.
- If mild diarrhea continues intermittently for over 1 week without obvious cause.
- If other symptoms of abdominal problems are present.
- For infants under 6 months old you should discuss *any* diarrhea problem with your health professional.
- If abdominal pain or severe discomfort accompanies diarrhea and is not immediately relieved by the passage of gas or diarrhea.

Food Poisoning

Two million Americans per year are victims of food poisoning. Most never know it. They attribute their symptoms of nausea, vomiting, diarrhea, and severe pain to a sudden case of stomach flu.

Bacteria are always present in the air and some always get to any food we eat. Fortunately, bacteria usually present no problem in themselves. However, at temperatures between 45° and 115°, the bacteria thrive and grow rapidly. They grow fastest on unrefrigerated meats and pastries (custards, whipped cream, etc.) and produce a poison or toxin which causes an acute inflammation of the intestines. The violence of the illness varies with the amount of toxin eaten and with individual susceptibility.

Most food poisoning occurs during the summer when picnickers eat unrefrigerated meats or on special occasions when cold cuts, turkey dressing, sauces, and other foods are not kept cold (under 45°). Other serious problems arise if foods are not prepared properly during home canning activities. If any bacteria survives the cooking, it may grow and produce toxin in the can or jar.

The symptoms of food poisoning do not begin immediately. From 3–36 hours may pass before the onset of the symptoms. Illness may last from 12 hours to as much as a week for common food poisoning.

Botulism, although rare, is fatal in 65% of cases. It is generally caused by improper home canning methods for low acid foods like beans or corn. Symptoms include blurred vision, inability to swallow, and progressive breathing difficulty.

PREVENTION

- Refrigerate meats to 40° or below.
- Be especially careful with large cooked meats like your holiday turkey, which require a long time to cool. Some parts of the meat may stay over 45° long enough to produce bacteria.
- Use a thermometer to check your refrigerator. It should be between 34° and 40°.
- Reheat meats to over 140° for 10 minutes to destroy bacteria before serving. Even then, the toxin may not be destroyed.
- Put party foods on ice to keep them cool during a party.
- Discard any cans or jars with bulging lids or leakage.
- Dispose of spoiled food so that it will not be eaten by humans or animals.
- Follow home canning and freezing instructions to the letter. Call your County Agricultural Extension office for advice.

HOME TREATMENT

- Nothing to eat or drink until vomiting has stopped. Ice chips and small sips of water are okay.

- Clear liquids only for 24 hours.
- Gradual progression to easily digestible foods.
- No spicy foods for 48 hours after all symptoms have gone.
- Check with others who may have eaten the same thing.
- Save a sample of the suspected food for analysis in case symptoms do not improve.

WHEN TO CALL A HEALTH PROFESSIONAL

- If you suspect food poisoning from a canned product or have any of the symptoms of botulism poisoning, call immediately. Take suspect food with you if you still have it.
- If you cannot control vomiting after 12 hours of ice chips-only treatment.
- If vital signs are not normal (temperature over 102°, respiration rate 4 breaths per minute above or below normal).
- If the victim appears very ill—especially in young children.

Gastroenteritis

Gastroenteritis is usually caused by a viral infection in the digestive sys-

tem. The infection brings on diarrhea to rid the intestines of irritants, and nausea or vomiting to
discourage eating until the problem
is cleared up. Although viral gastroenteritis (stomach flu) will usually go away on its own within
24–48 hours, your own home care
may shorten the time to recovery
and lessen the chance of complications.

Bacterial infections such as dys-
entery or salmonella food poisoning can also cause gastroenteritis.
Excesses of alcohol or food may
also be the culprits.

Symptoms of the infection include back and muscle aches, abdominal pain, headaches, and fever.

HOME TREATMENT

- No food or drink for several hours. Ice chips and
  small sips of water are
  okay.
- Clear liquids only for 24
  hours. Start with a few sips
  at a time.
- Go through the home physical exam, page 3, and
  read through the abdominal pain section of this
  chapter, page 26. Record
  your observations.
- Bed rest until aches subside.
- Soups, mild foods and liquids only on second day
  and until all symptoms are
  gone for 48 hours.

- Return to regular diet several days after symptoms
  have stopped.

NOTE: Infants and small children can dehydrate very quickly
with fluid loss from both vomiting
and diarrhea. See Dehydration,
page 30. Infants should be taken off
all fluids until vomiting is controlled
—up to 4 hours.

WHEN TO CALL A HEALTH PROFESSIONAL

- If vomiting and diarrhea
  are violent or if patient is
  weakened by age (very old
  or very young) or by other
  health problems.
- If diarrhea is bloody or
  very black.
- If vomiting continues off
  and on for over 12 hours
  without improvement. (2–6
  hours for small children.)
- If violent retching continues for over 2 hours.
- If temperature of 102° or
  higher persists.
- Severe, increasing, or con-
  tinuing pain in abdomen
  for over 4 hours.
- Mild but continuous pain
  lasting over 12 hours.
- If diarrhea continues after
  48 hours of liquids-only
  diet.
- If signs of dehydration appear, see Dehydration on
  page 30.

Indigestion

Indigestion is any irritation of the stomach lining. It is often caused by excessive consumption of alcohol or spicy foods. Emotional tension and hurried eating also contribute to indigestion. Usual symptoms include a burning sensation an hour or so after eating and reduced appetite. Acute indigestion may cause a feeling of fullness and pressure in the stomach, nausea or vomiting. Continual indigestion often precedes the development of ulcers.

HOME TREATMENT

- Reduce strength of stomach acids by eating bland foods such as cream soups, potatoes, or breads, drinking milk and taking antacids. Drink more fluids, but not coffee or other stimulants.
- Relax at mealtime. Eat more slowly. Try to lie down after a meal when possible.
- Review symptoms and treatment of ulcers, page 38.

WHEN TO CALL A HEALTH PROFESSIONAL

- If indigestion discomfort increases enough to suggest ulcer formation. See Ulcers, page 38.
- If indigestion-like discomfort is accompanied by other symptoms, such as shortness of breath, which might suggest heart problems. See Chest Pain, page 149.

Pinworms

Pinworms are small thin parasites that commonly infect the digestive tracts of young children. Pinworms are most common in 4- to 6-year-olds although any aged child may be infected. The worms live in the upper end of the large intestine, near the appendix, and must travel to the outside of the anus to lay their eggs. The egg laying almost always occurs at night and usually causes the child to scratch the anal area. Then, when the child later sucks a thumb or licks a finger, the eggs are ingested and the cycle begins again.

The symptoms of pinworms vary with the degree of infection. Severe cases can cause acute abdominal pain. More common symptoms include the loss of appetite and occasional diarrhea. Signs of itching in the anal area are the surest clues.

If you suspect pinworms, it's easy to find out for sure in your own home and at no cost. Go into your child's darkened bedroom several hours after bedtime. Shine a flashlight on the anus. The light will cause the tiny thread-like worms to start back into the anus. If you don't see the worms after checks on 2 or 3 nights, it is unlikely that the child is infected.

Remember, pinworms will hit most American families at one time or another. Most never realize it. Alert parents can watch for the signs of pinworms and limit their effect on the health of their growing children.

HOME TREATMENT

- Ask your pharmacist for a non-prescription vermifuge (drug) effective against pinworms. P.W. Tabs are often used.
- Treat every child in the house between the ages of 2 and 10. If infection recurs, you may wish to treat the entire family.
- Check the infected child several nights after the treatment using the flashlight. If worms are still present a more powerful prescription vermifuge may be needed.
- Improve all cleanliness practices in the household.
  - o Trim and keep short all fingernails.
  - o Require frequent hand washing.
  - o Sanitize toilet area with a strong disinfectant cleaner.
  - o Wash all bedding and sanitize bed area.
  - o Require morning shower, daily change of pajamas and underwear.

WHEN TO CALL A HEALTH PROFESSIONAL

- If use of any drug produces adverse reactions such as vomiting or increased pain.
- If you suspect pinworms but the nighttime checks find nothing. A health professional can do a number of lab tests to diagnose pinworms. These tests are not highly reliable, however, and may require several return visits.
- If you are not able to eliminate the pinworms with the non-prescription drug, a health professional can prescribe a stronger, more effective drug.

Ulcers

An ulcer is a break in the inside lining of the gastrointestinal tract. Ulcers are formed at the lower end of the esophagus, in the stomach, or most frequently, in the duodenum (the first part of the small intestine).

Every stomach produces strong acids and other potent gastric juices in order to digest food. Under emotional stress or tension our bodies tend to produce more acids than are needed for digestion. This excess acid may begin to burn through the protective mucus which coats the stomach or intestinal wall.

Symptoms of an ulcer may include a burning pain, gas, vomiting, or belching. The burning pain is usually strongest when the stomach is empty. Ulcer patients are sometimes awakened by pain in the middle of the night. A glass of milk or a piece of bread will usually relieve that pain by neutralizing the acid for a while.

as possible. Avoid spicy foods and drink milk frequently.

- When you first suspect you have an ulcer, try to heal it quickly. By taking a few days to relax and concentrate on a more soothing diet, you may well avoid an expensive hospitalization.

HOME TREATMENT

- Slow down. Ulcers are difficult to heal if emotional stress and tension continue to pour more acid into the system. The suggestions on page 200 may help you deal with stress.
- Antacids are usually necessary to neutralize your gastric acids long enough for the ulcer to heal. You need frequent and large amounts of antacids to do the job. Talk to your health professional about how much to take. Non-absorbable antacids like Maalox, Mylanta, or Gelusil are best. Most antacids have high salt contents and should be used with caution by persons on low-sodium diets.
- Change your diet. Eliminate alcohol and reduce coffee, tea, and carbonated drinks to absolute minimums. Eat more often. Schedule 4–6 light meals over the day to keep the acids neutralized as much

WHEN TO CALL A HEALTH PROFESSIONAL

- To diagnose and evaluate a suspected ulcer. An examination, history, and tests can often determine the presence, location, and severity of an ulcer.
- To determine appropriate antacid dosage.
- If vomiting accompanies pain.
- If severe pain is not relieved by your treatment program.
- If patient appears unusually weak or pale.

Urinary Tract Infections

Urinary tract infections are frequent and annoying problems. Early symptoms are a burning sensation during urination, itching, or pain in the urethra (tube through which urine is expelled from the bladder).

Urinary infections are usually caused by bacteria which are normally present in the digestive system. Because of the closeness between the anus and the urethra in women, they are much more susceptible than are men to the infection. Any mild irritation to the vaginal area may increase the likelihood of urinary infection. Vaginal douches, sexual intercourse, or even the ingestion of alcohol or spicy food may contribute to the problem.

Most urinary tract infections can be eliminated by home treatment methods in about 3 days. Untreated, some infections may go on to infect the kidneys and cause permanent kidney problems. Because of this danger, pain upon urination should always be treated promptly.

PREVENTION

- Women should wipe from front to back after going to the toilet. This will reduce the bacteria spread from the rectum to the vagina.
- Women should avoid excessive douching or use of vaginal deodorants.
- Drink more fluids—water is best.
- Women susceptible to urinary infections should urinate before and after intercourse. Drinking extra water after intercourse may also help prevent infection.

HOME TREATMENT

- Examine vagina and check temperature twice daily.

See home physical exam, page 3.
- Drink lots of fluids to wash out the infection.
- Avoid alcohol, coffee, and spicy foods.
- If abdominal pain or vaginal burning and redness occur in a young girl, consider the possibility of an allergy to bubble bath or other cleaning aid.
- Get extra rest.

WHEN TO CALL A HEALTH PROFESSIONAL

- When pain on urination is accompanied by any of the following symptoms:
  o Chills and/or fever over 101°
  o A frequent inability to urinate when you feel the urge
  o Pain or tenderness in the thighs
  o Backaches
  o Bloody urine
  o Nausea or vomiting
- If there is any history of kidney infections.
- If pain on urination has not diminished after 3 days of home treatment.
- A health professional will usually examine the urinary tract opening and may culture a urine sample to determine the kind of bacteria present. Although the culture report may take sev-

Types of Vaginitis

TYPE	SYMPTOMS
Yeast or monilia	White, curdy discharge like cottage cheese, burning on urination, itching. May cause skin rash on thighs and vulva.
Trichomonas	Severe itching, pain, and profuse yellow-green frothy discharge with a foul odor.
Non-specific or bacteria	Itching, discharge and sour odor.

eral days, the patient may be given antibiotic medication immediately depending on the severity of the symptoms. If antibiotics are prescribed, be sure to take them for the full period prescribed (about 10 days) even if you feel better after only 2 or 3 days. The bacteria may become resistant if not completely eliminated. Call your health professional if a rash appears or you think there is any other adverse reaction to the drug.

Vaginitis

Vaginitis is any vaginal infection or inflammation characterized by a change in vaginal discharge. Healthy women have a small amount of odorless, non-irritating discharge. The amount varies from woman to woman and may increase in certain times of the menstrual cycle. General symptoms of vaginitis are a marked change from the normal discharge, sometimes accompanied by itching, burning on urination, and pain during intercourse. Listed below are 3 types of vaginitis and their symptoms.

These 3 types are caused by organisms that are normally found in the vagina along with other protective bacteria. The vagina usually has a slightly acid pH (the measure of acidity and alkalinity) which resists infection. If something happens to upset the balance of bacteria or the usual pH, vaginitis can result. Four ways for this to happen are:

- *Excessive* douching which allows the other organisms to take over after washing away the protective bacteria. Too much douching may also upset the vaginal pH.
- The use of antibiotics may kill the protective bacteria.

- Infectious organisms may be introduced through sexual intercourse.
- Tension can change the hormonal balance and upset the normal vagina.

Vaginitis is common and is not necessarily a venereal disease. It is not very serious and some women seem more susceptible than others. An aggravating fact about vaginitis is that it can recur.

PREVENTION

- Wear cotton underpants. The organisms which cause vaginitis grow best in warm, moist places, and nylon underwear and pantyhose retain heat and perspiration. Avoid pants that are tight in the crotch and thighs.
- Avoid douching frequently.
  A healthy vagina will clean itself.
- It is sometimes possible to prevent bacterial vaginitis by eating yogurt or buttermilk while taking antibiotics.

HOME TREATMENT

- A bacterial or non-specific vaginitis *may* go away by itself in 3–4 days.
- A mild yeast infection may be cured by a mild vinegar douche. Use 2 tablespoons white vinegar per quart of water. This will help restore an acid pH in the vagina.
- Avoid using feminine deodorant sprays, as they may cause more irritation.
- Avoid scratching.
- Abstain from sex until the infection is cleared. Although the infection does not usually cause symptoms in men, you may become reinfected later by your sex partner if he has the germs.
- If you need to see a health professional, do not douche before the appointment since it may make diagnosis difficult.

WHEN TO CALL A HEALTH PROFESSIONAL

- If you recognize a yeast infection and it is mild, then try the vinegar douche. Otherwise, see a health professional for any symptoms of vaginitis. A lab test will identify the organism causing the infection.
- Antibiotics can be prescribed to clear up the infection. See page 227, which describes appropriate use of antibiotics.

Vomiting

Vomiting is any rejection of stomach or intestinal contents. Although vomiting can be a symptom of a large number of moderate and serious diseases, most vomiting is due to a variety of relatively minor problems that are readily treatable at home.

HOME TREATMENT

- Nothing by mouth for 4 hours. Small ice chips and small sips of water may be all right.
- Clear liquids only for 24 hours. Start with a few sips at a time.
- Go through the home physical exam, page 3.
- Bed rest until aches subside.
- Soups, mild foods and liquids only on second day and until all symptoms are gone for 48 hours.
- Return to regular diet several days after symptoms have stopped.

WHEN TO CALL A HEALTH PROFESSIONAL

- If vomiting is severe or "violent." (It shoots out in large quantities.)
- If vomiting does not stop after 12 hours of the suggested treatment. (2–6 hours for small children.)
- If violent retching continues for over 2 hours.
- If there is blood in the vomit.
- If signs of dehydration appear, see discussion on dehydration, page 30.
- If abdominal pain is severe or constant and does not seem to be relieved by the passage of gas or stools. Although discomfort and cramping often accompany vomiting, other pain may signal more serious problems. Your health professional should be called if there is any doubt regarding the type, severity, or cause of the pain.

3

Backaches

Back pain is one of the most common complaints people have about their health and accounts for over 18 million visits to doctors each year. Nearly all backaches are caused by inadequate exercise, awkward or heavy lifting, poor posture, mental stress, or improper sleeping positions. At least 9 out of 10 backaches can be prevented, even if you start late.

Most troublesome back pain is located in the lower back. There the lumbar vertebrae must support the entire weight of the upper body. The back consists of the spine (the vertebrae or bones), the discs which separate each bone, and the muscles and ligaments which hold everything together and allow movement.

If the back muscles are not kept in good shape, 3 things can happen and they all hurt. First, the muscles can be stretched too far and "strained." Like any strained muscle, a back muscle must be rested for quite a while to recover from a strain. Second, the ligaments can be stretched too far or "sprained." Ligaments are tough bands of tissue that connect bones together. When they are sprained or torn they cause great pain and also must be rested in order to heal. The third problem area is the disc. Spinal discs are very strong and filled with a resilient jelly-like substance. They act like shock absorbers to protect the bones from hitting each other. When discs are continually abused by stress which the back muscles can't handle, they get brittle and crack or rupture. Further abuse can squeeze the jelly material out through the crack. As the jelly presses on the nerves in the spinal column, it causes severe pain in the back and frequently down the legs. This condition, which limits movement and causes a "stiff" back, is often called a "slipped disc." Usually, however, the disc is ruptured or flattened but is rarely slipped as the term implies.

The 3 problems of muscles, ligaments, and discs are related. When the muscles and ligaments are not overloaded, they protect the discs. Only when they become stretched or weakened is the disc abused.

Unfortunately, too few people know how to protect their backs. By age 20, many millions of Americans have at least 1 ruptured disc. All such persons are subject to back pain even though they have not yet experienced any discomfort. They can avoid future back pain only if they treat their backs with more respect and a little common sense.

The remainder of this chapter is divided into 2 sections. The first deals with how to avoid back pain. Simple exercise suggestions and lifting posture tips are presented. The second section deals with treating both minor and severe back pain. Although 90% of backaches can be cared for at home, they are never a welcome occurrence. If you carefully follow the directions in the first section, you may never need to study the second.

Back Pain Prevention

The objective in back pain prevention is to reduce the lower curve or "hollow" in the back to a minimum. The greater the curve in the lower spine, the greater the pressure on the back-most portion of each disc. Continual pinching of the disc causes it to weaken and crack.

There are 2 basic ways to reduce the hollow in the back. One is to strengthen the abdominal and buttocks muscles. The other is to reduce the stresses on the discs by improved posture and lifting habits. The abdominal muscles oppose the back muscles in keeping the spine straight. When they become weakened, the strong back muscles begin to shorten and force the spine into a curved position. As the weakened abdomen sags, it also pulls the spine forward, increasing the curve and the pressure on the back of the disc. Weakened buttocks muscles also tend to increase the hollow of the back. Simple exercises to strengthen these muscles are illustrated in this chapter.

Posture Tips to Save Your Back

Most Americans have been taught since childhood to *stand up straight*. Unfortunately, this can be grossly exaggerated. If you try to stand up too straight, with your chest out and your shoulders back, your lower back may suffer. A more appropriate commandment for parents to teach their children is to *keep your lower back straight*. As you shall see, it makes quite a difference.

Throughout this section are illustrated correct and incorrect postures for sitting, standing, driving, sleeping, and gardening. In every

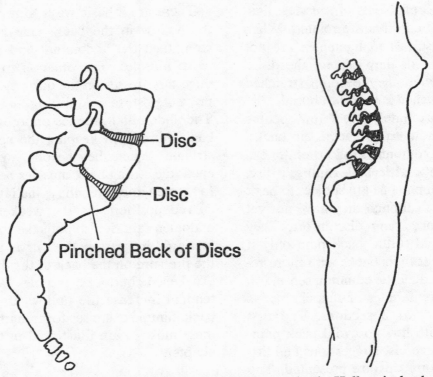

Pressure on discs from increased hollow in low back. Hollow in back causes backbone to pinch back edge of disc.

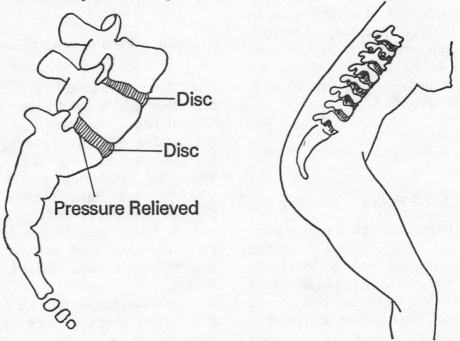

When hollow is eliminated the pressure is distributed evenly over the disc.

case the rule is the same: eliminate the hollow in the lower back. If you spend a lot of time each day doing any of these activities wrong, your back may be suffering whether you have felt it yet or not. Fortunately, many of these tips require little effort to adopt. They do, however, require your constant attention, at least until they have replaced the back-breaking habits you may now have. To adopt other tips on a regular basis, you may have to strengthen your abdominal muscles using the exercises suggested on pages 53–55.

SITTING

Always sit with your back rounded to eliminate the hollow in the low back. Some stodgy etiquette experts may call that "slumping." It is, however, the correct position if you expect to ease or avoid low back pain.

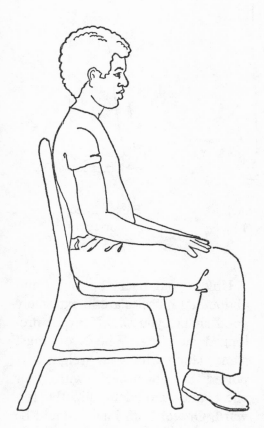

This is incorrect.

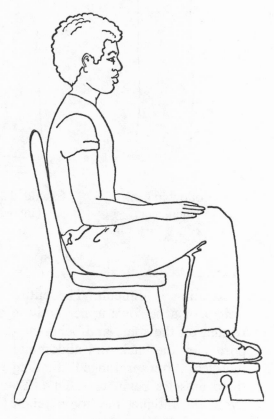

This is correct.
Keep knees higher than hips by using a foot rest or a shorter chair.

Standing postures

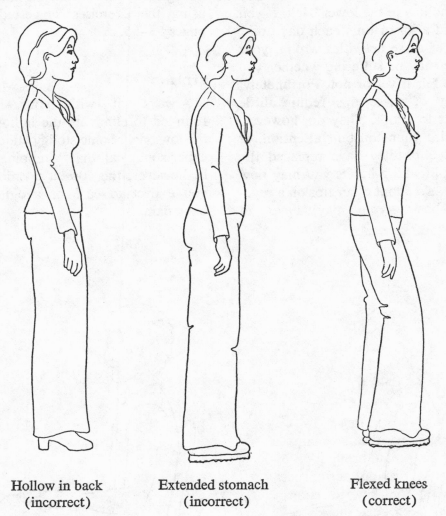

Hollow in back   Extended stomach   Flexed knees
(incorrect)   (incorrect)   (correct)

STANDING

Standing is difficult. The entire weight of a person's upper body is resting on the spine and being supported by the back and abdominal muscles. After prolonged standing these muscles begin to fatigue. To avoid the fatigue, the body weight is shifted backward to rest more weight on the spine or lower vertebrae.

Unless your back, buttocks, and abdominal muscles are in extremely good shape, you should avoid prolonged standing. When you must stand, stand with your weight supported by your heels with your chest and shoulders slightly forward. One or both knees should be slightly bent or flexed. Standing in high heels is particularly troublesome for the lower back.

Driving postures

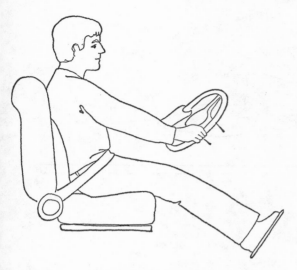

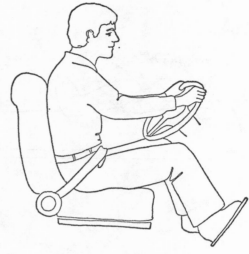

This is incorrect.

This is correct.
Keep knees higher than hips.

DRIVING

Driving posture tips are really no different than those for sitting. However, because so many people suffer back pain brought on by long car rides, driving merits special attention. The key to comfortable driving is to keep the knees higher than the hips. This stretches the spine and relieves the pressure on the discs. Keep this in mind when you select a car. Knee room should be much more important than how far the seat slides back. For greatest back comfort the seat should be as far forward as possible without interfering with steering. On long drives, stop often for roadside rests and back exercises. The squat-bounce shown on page 58 may give considerable relief.

SLEEPING

The most comfortable sleeping position for most people is on the side with knees drawn up. Sleeping on the back with a pillow under the knees also puts the spine at rest.

Never sleep on your stomach. It exaggerates the hollow in the low back and is a frequent cause of low back pain. Lying flat on the back without the knees propped can also cause problems.

A firm bed is quite helpful to a painful back. The mattress should be soft enough for comfort and blood circulation but should be supported by a very firm or hard base. Placing a ½-inch sheet of plywood between a mattress and a sagging box spring has restored the useful life of many beds.

Sleeping positions

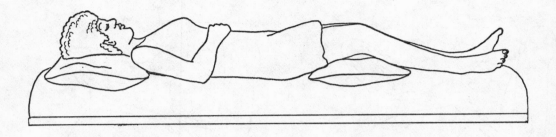

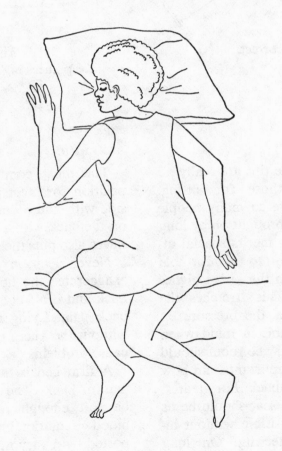

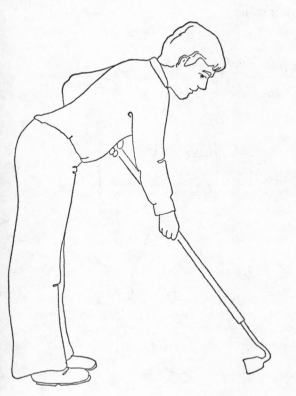

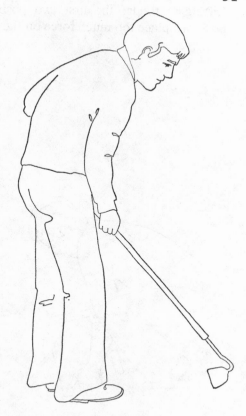

Incorrect   Correct

MOPPING, IRONING, WORKING, ETC.

Backaches are often brought on by mopping, ironing, working over a low work bench, hoeing a garden, or shaving over a sink, activities which normally require the weight to be shifted forward. This strains the low back muscles since they must be in constant use to keep the body from falling over. Actually, the lower back is usually bent backward in such activities (again pinching the disc) with all of the forward bending coming from the hips.

You can avoid back pain from these activities. Just follow the postures illustrated above. Try them yourself. Notice that when one foot is placed in front and the knees are bent, the hollow of the back is eliminated. Also, by placing one foot on a step stool or support, the pain from ironing or shaving can be avoided.

Lifting methods: the first two positions here are correct, while the other positions place too much force on the lower spine.

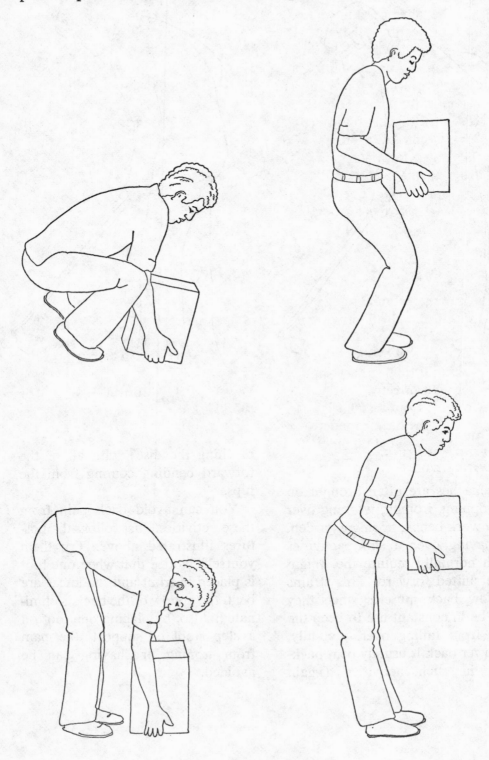

Lifting Tips to Save Your Back

Heavy or awkward lifting greatly increases the damage done to the discs by poor posture. Heavy lifting done using the incorrect methods shown on page 52 at bottom places a tremendous crushing force on the discs of the lower spine. Discs cannot hold up forever under such abuse and their weakening will eventually cause low back pain.

Notice that in the correct lift the spine is not erect, but slightly slumped. At least one foot should be flat on the floor to avoid the unstable tiptoe stance. The lifting should be done with the legs, not the back.

Remember to eliminate the hollow in the back at all times, even when lifting a very small object.

The following rules should be followed during lifting or carrying activities:

1. Always lift from a squatting position with the back rounded and at least one foot flat on the floor.
2. If you have a pen in your breast pocket and it falls out while you are lifting, then you are lifting incorrectly.
3. Never lift a heavy load above the waist.
4. Carry loads at waist level with hips and knees bent.

Exercises to Save Your Back

Exercise can be the most important part in the prevention of back pain. This section illustrates 5 exercises that can help prevent or control low back pain. Although the exercises are a good idea for everyone, they are a must for those who are prone to back problems. Those with already diagnosed disc problems should discuss the advisability of such exercises with a health professional.

Each exercise plays a different role in strengthening and toning abdominal, back, and buttocks muscles. Each should be done 6–25 times per session depending on physical ability. Two sessions per day are recommended. It shouldn't take more than 5 minutes per session. The exercises are given in the order of less strenuous ones for limbering up to more strenuous.

EXERCISE 1: BACKFLATTENING

This is perhaps the easiest and most relaxing of all the exercises. It works on the abdominal, buttocks, and back muscles at the same time.

Have your feet and shoulders flat on the floor, body relaxed. Pull the stomach muscles in, pinch buttocks together—feel the low back flatten down against floor. Hold for count of 5, relax and repeat.

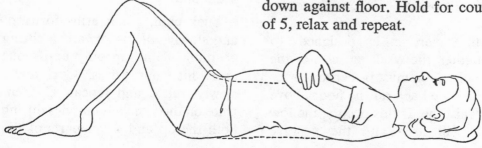

Backflattening exercise

EXERCISE 2: KNEES TO CHEST

The purpose of this exercise is to stretch the strong, short back muscles and to restore a full range of forward movement to the vertebrae of the low back.

This exercise affords more relief for your back than any of the others described. For this reason many persons perform this exercise first since it helps relieve back stiffness and soreness and enables them to do the rest of the exercises with less discomfort.

Hold up both knees as shown. Pull knees gently toward armpits. Keep knees apart. Keep head and shoulders on the floor. Relax arms to original position and repeat.

EXERCISE 3: BUTTOCKS LIFT

Lie flat on your back with your knees bent and heels 4–8 inches from your buttocks and a pillow under your head. Firmly contract the muscles of the buttocks, lifting the buttocks as high off the mat or floor as possible. Hold the contracted position for a second and then slowly relax, allowing the buttocks to ease back down to their original position. Repeat the exercise.

This exercise is designed to strengthen the weak muscles of the buttocks. You must be certain never to raise the back off the floor above the waistline. If this occurs, the low back will arch and the positive value of the exercise will be negated.

EXERCISE 4: BACK STRETCHING

Sit on the floor with your legs fully extended and relaxed and your upper body straight. Your head will be tilted forward.

Bend the upper body slowly and smoothly forward in an attempt to touch your toes.

Return to an upright position and repeat the exercise. Make certain the upper body is never bent backward beyond a straight sitting position.

This exercise also stretches the strong, short back muscles and helps to restore and maintain a full range of forward movement in the low back.

Exercise 4 should never be done by a person who is experiencing pain in the back of the leg. This is because the exercise stretches the sciatic nerve to the legs and thus would increase the pain. The exercise should, however, be started as soon as the leg pain subsides.

EXERCISE 5: MODIFIED SITS UPS

Tuck chin, reach arms forward, and slowly *roll* up toward a sitting position. Come up only until your arms hit your knees. Curl down slowly, relax, and repeat. Concentrate on the stomach muscles during both the up and down parts of the

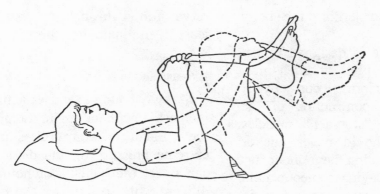

Knees to chest exercise

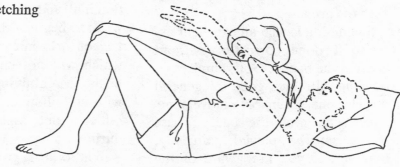

Buttocks lift

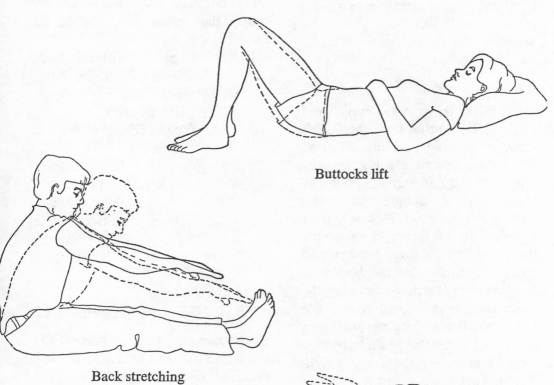

Back stretching

Modified sit up

exercise. Avoid jerking the body up.

This exercise is designed to develop the little-used stomach muscles. When performed correctly, it causes a firm contraction of the abdominal or "stomach" muscles alone. You should never anchor your feet by placing them under furniture or by having someone hold them. This increases the hollow in the low back. Extending the legs with the knees straight also increases the hollow and should be avoided with sit ups.

GENERAL EXERCISE

Hiking, biking, swimming, and other activities that keep the body's muscles in good tone are all good preventive exercises for a healthy back. Jogging, however, is not recommended for people who suffer from low back pain. Not only does it provide unnecessary "jogs" to the damaged discs, but the tendency to jog erect emphasizes the hollow in the low back, further damaging the discs. Bicycle riding can provide the same benefits as jogging but keeps the back in a restful position by supporting much of the body weight with the arms.

Swimming is also an excellent exercise if done correctly (without arching the back). Golf, tennis, and bowling, although good for general muscle tone, all involve movements which can arch the back. These sports can be played painlessly, however, if you are aware of the motions to avoid and alter your

serve, follow-through, or ball release to eliminate disc abuse.

EXERCISES TO AVOID

Many common exercises actually increase low back pain. Some of these ill-conceived exercises place extreme pressure on the discs and can offset the benefits of hours of diligent work to improve the back. The following exercises are potentially harmful since they can increase the hollow, and should be avoided.

AVOID: Legs up (lifting both legs in an extended position while lying on your back).

Weight lifting above the waist.

Any exercise which involves bending backward while standing.

Arching the back while lying on the stomach.

Straight leg sit ups.

Exercises and Pregnancy

Pregnancy puts added stress on the back muscles and spine. If the abdominal and buttocks muscles are weak to begin with, pregnancy may trigger chronic back problems which will not be cured by childbirth. Maintaining good posture with no hollow in the lower back is difficult but especially important during pregnancy, because the weight of the growing fetus pulls the abdomen forward. Exercises

1–5 or similar exercises recommended by the woman's health professional are the best ways to help your back in pregnancy. The exercises should begin early in pregnancy (if not before) and should be continued into the ninth month. They should then be resumed several days after delivery under the supervision of your health professional. One out of every 5 pregnant women suffer back discomfort before or after delivery. A carefully planned and responsibly followed exercise program can eliminate or greatly reduce the discomfort.

Treatment of Back Pain

When you get a backache the first thing to do is to try to determine its type and cause. Ask yourself the questions here.

You may wish to go through the home physical exam procedures in Chapter 1 to get an overall view of your own health other than the back pains.

Once you have narrowed down the pain's most probable cause you are ready to attack the problem.

TENSION AND FATIGUE BACKACHES

If the pain seems to be mostly due to tension and/or poor posture during back-tiring activities, warm, relaxing baths and gentle massaging can help eliminate the pain. Rest your back in positions which reduce the pain. Elevating your feet on a chair with your knees bent while lying on your back is very relaxing. The exercise program discussed earlier should also be tried. Exercises 1 and 2 are particularly helpful and easy to do. See page 202 for a discussion of how to reduce tension in your life.

STRAINS, SPRAINS, AND DISC PAIN

Muscle strains and sprained ligaments are usually caused by a sudden bending of the spine, especially when the back is tense or tired. Awkward lifting or a fall or twist may cause the muscles and ligaments to stretch too far. One or

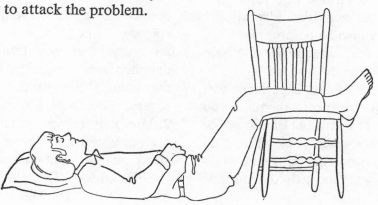

Back resting position

Back Pain: History and Exam

Is the ache in the upper or lower back?

Has there been a blow or sudden injury to the back?

Could tension have contributed to the back pain?

Have prolonged activities been performed using the pain-producing postures discussed earlier (sitting, standing, working, jogging, etc.) without eliminating the hollow in the lower back?

Have you strained or sprained muscles or ligaments through awkward movements?

Have you experienced any sharp pain in either leg together with the back pain?

Are there other symptoms of illness that might be related to the back pain?

---

more of the vertebral discs may also have been pressured by the movement. If so, a shooting pain in the leg may be felt.

When you first feel a catch or slip in the back there are 2 things you can do to avoid or reduce the expected pain. First, as soon as you feel the pain, go into a flat-footed squat and bounce up and down *gently* 15–20 times as shown in the illustration.

Each bounce should be no more than 2–3 inches. Rest and repeat the series several times before resuming your activities. Exercises 1 and 2 may also be helpful just after the slip is felt, especially if the pain is too great for the bounce.

If because of past experience you are still worried about the pain, you may wish to put a cold pack or ice bag on the lower back. The cold will help reduce the pain and swelling and may avoid the muscle spasm.

Although cold packs and the

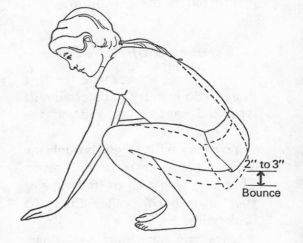

2" to 3"

Bounce

Low back pain bounce

bounce can often prevent an acute episode of low back pain, they don't always work at once. Use your own common sense to judge how often they should be repeated for the next several days. Add Exercises 1 and 2. Use pain relievers sensibly. Moderate use of aspirin combined with good resting positions can reduce the discomfort. Complete masking of the pain might allow movement that would further injure the back.

If the strain was a bad one and the pain remains for over 2 days, you should substitute warm baths and heating pads for the ice packs. For the greatest comfort, rest in bed on your back with your knees propped up on pillows and with a pillow under your head. Exercise 1 should be repeated every few hours during the hours that you are awake.

If the pain has not subsided after 4–5 days of bed rest, you should consult your health professional. Usually by that time you should be able to get up an hour at a time and gradually return to the full exercise program. You should be able to resume normal activities after 8–10 days of the suggested treatment.

HOME TREATMENT

- Immediately upon feeling slip:
  o Buttocks bounce exercise and/or Exercises 1 and 2.
  o Ice packs.
- During first 24–48 hours:
  o Repeat exercises every few hours.
  o Cold packs for first 24 hours.
  o Rest on back with knees propped.
  o Pain relievers should be used sensibly. Use the *minimum* needed to allow relaxation in the back-rest position.
- After 48 hours:
  o Continue Exercises 1 and 2.
  o Gradually add other exercises.
  o Substitute warm baths and heating pads for cold packs.
  o Continue resting back until symptoms subside.

WHEN TO CALL A HEALTH PROFESSIONAL

- When severe back pain results from an accident or blow to the back. *DO NOT MOVE AN ACCIDENT VICTIM WHO MAY HAVE AN INJURED SPINE.*
- When severe disabling pain suddenly occurs in the leg and foot *without* significant cause.
- If substantial relief for a sprain, strain, or disc injury is not obtained within 5 days of recommended home treatment.
- Pain in the back is not always due to problems of the muscles and bones of the back. Abdominal or pelvic disorders may also cause back pain. Back pains from such disorders often foretell a very serious condition. Although the great majority of back pains come from the back problems discussed earlier, back pain can be caused by

problems with the following organs:

o Kidneys—The kidneys sit right up against the back. Kidney infections can produce back pain.

o Urinary, Bladder—Although located in the lower front portion of the abdomen, bladder infections can produce back pain because the same nerves serve the bladder and the back.

o Prostate Gland—The prostate gland is a part of the male reproductive system and is located below the bladder. When infected, it too can cause low back pain.

o Female Genitals—Inflammation of the uterus or ovaries may cause severe back pain. Normal menstrual pain is often felt in the back as well.

o Intestines—Infections of the intestines such as the stomach flu can cause back pain.

If you notice any other symptoms which might suggest any of the above disorders in connection with a backache, call a health professional.

Low back pain sufferers often will want to see a health professional during acute episodes of back pain. Unfortunately, there is little a physician can do. Muscle relaxants are sometimes prescribed to eliminate the muscle spasm pain. However, ice and proper muscle relaxation positions can usually do an equally effective job. If muscle relaxants are used, care should be taken not to reinjure the unprotected parts of the back. Since the trip to and from a health professional's office can be very painful and even harmful to your back, carefully consider the merits of home treatment first.

4

Headaches

Any number of things can cause headaches. Most are minor and most headaches will go away in time. However, headaches hurt and most of us want to know how to get rid of the pain and how to prevent its return.

With just a little detective work it is possible to trace the cause of many headaches. While there is no definite pattern to link *where* it hurts to *why* it hurts, there are certain questions to ask which may give clues to potential causes. Page 62 lists these questions and some potential headache causes.

Headache pain can occur anywhere on the head. Most headaches occur when the muscles of the head or neck become tense and contract, causing the blood vessels of the head to go into spasm. This change in the flow of blood to the head is the cause of pain.

Too many people treat headaches lightly. "A couple of aspirin and it'll be gone soon." It is important to remember that a headache is a symptom that all is not well in the body. Whether the cause is a serious organic disease, or simply tension, pollution, or hay fever, you should take time to try to determine that cause. With just a little effort, you can usually discover a reasonable cause and perhaps prevent future headaches.

By far, most headaches are caused by tension or stress in our lives. These are headaches the individual can most easily control.

Rarely, headache will be a sign of a serious illness. If you are bothered by persistent severe headaches which have no cause you can discover, or if any of the following occur, you should see a health professional:

- Sudden onset of pain without a specific cause. If pain wakes you in the middle of the night, or you know exactly what you were doing when the pain struck, that is a sudden pain.

- High fever of 103° and headache with no other symptoms.
- A stiff neck, fever and headache are danger signals of meningitis. Test to see that person can touch chin to chest, mouth shut, without pain.
- Headache and confusion

not following an injury. Confusion is common following an injury.

- Headache accompanied by loss of coordination, double vision, or other neurological symptoms.
- Recurring headaches in children.
- Headaches of increasing frequency and severity.

CLUES TO POTENTIAL HEADACHE CAUSES

- Does the headache occur on rising? The culprit may be sinus or allergy trouble. Humidifying the bedroom may ease this problem. Sinus headache can worsen in the afternoon.
- Does the headache precede the menstrual period each month? It may be caused by pre-menstrual tension.
- Does the headache occur each afternoon or evening, This may be a sign of eyestrain. Rest your eyes and have your vision checked.
- Does the headache occur an hour or so before mealtime? Hunger is a frequent cause of headache.
- Is there a sharp pain directly behind the eye? This can be a sign of glaucoma, a serious eye disease, and should be checked by a health professional.
- Is the headache just on one side? This is a clue to migraine, discussed on page 64.
- Does the headache regularly follow any activity or event? May be a tension headache. These headaches are described on page 63.
- Did you over-indulge in alcohol the night before a headache? Hangovers are all too frequent, and unpleasant. Coffee may help by constricting dilated blood vessels in the head. Prevent the next one!
- Are you taking any new medication? Some medications cause severe headaches in susceptible people.
- Smoking too much can cause headaches.
- Pollution can cause headaches.
- Hay fever and allergies sometimes cause headaches.
- Headaches also accompany other illnesses, such as colds and flu.

Otherwise, you can usually discover the cause of a headache and ease the pain simply, at home.

It is important to stress that aspirin is not a cure-all for headaches. Occasionally aspirin masks symptoms that might aid a faster diagnosis of an ailment. Also, continued overuse of aspirin may lead to aspirin poisoning.

Tension Headaches

About 90% of all headaches are caused by tension. Anyone can get a tension headache, not just the "nervous type." Tension headaches are often caused by the tightening of the muscles of the back and shoulders.

A tension headache may occur as pain all over the head, as a feeling of pressure, or as a band around the head. Some people feel a dull pressing burning feeling above the eyes. Rarely can you pinpoint the center or source of pain.

PREVENTION

- For tension headaches particularly, the best cure is prevention. Often you can relate your headache to a recent activity which caused tension: grocery shopping, a meeting, or paying the bills. The elimination of the cause is the best prevention, but that is often impossible. In those cases just knowing some event makes you tense and taking time before and after the event to relax may help.

HOME TREATMENT

You should avoid frequent use of aspirin, acetaminophen, or other stronger pain killers because they can mask the pain and prevent you from eliminating the source of your headaches. However, aspirin or acetaminophen may relieve a tension headache. Be sure if you take them to take the appropriate dosage. Aspirin is an irritant to the stomach lining and should be used with caution if the headache is accompanied by an upset or nervous stomach.

Simpler cures are:

- Try to stop whatever you are doing and just close your eyes and sit. Exhale and inhale slowly and deeply.
- Lie down in a darkened room with a cool cloth on your forehead.
- Try to relax the head and neck muscles.
- Apply heat with a heating pad or hot water bottle or take a hot shower.
- Massage the neck muscles. Massage gently, firmly, toward the heart.
- Try a relaxation exercise:

Imagine that your neck muscles are loose, that your head is balanced at the end of your spine, and if you tip your head just slightly, it will fall in that direction. Let your mouth fall open, jaw relaxed. Close your eyes. Relax the forehead muscles. Now imagine a hole in your head, and inhale and exhale slowly. As you exhale imagine that the pain is flowing out of that hole. This will take some time and concentration. It is not an instant cure, but a good one.

- Either vigorous or isometric exercise helps relieve tension for some people.
- Good ways to cope with stress begin on page 200.

WHEN TO CALL A HEALTH PROFESSIONAL

- If unexplained headaches occur more than 3–5 times a week.
- If a headache is of very sudden onset.
- If a headache is very severe and cannot be relieved with the above measures.
- If you need help discovering and/or eliminating the source of your tension headaches. Often talking it over with a health professional is helpful.

Migraine Headaches

Migraine headaches are a specific kind of headache with specific symptoms. They occur less frequently than most people think. No one is sure exactly why migraine headaches occur in some people, but recent research has given hope that those with migraines may be able to learn to prevent them.

It is important to remember that severity is not the only symptom of a migraine. Tension headaches can be quite painful but can never become migraines.

The pain of a migraine headache is caused by the increased dilation or widening of the blood vessels in the head. Sometimes you can see the arteries at the temples throbbing during an episode.

The person who experiences migraine headaches often has relatives who have had the headaches. They are frequently fast-moving, tense, and active people. Migraines occur more frequently in women than in men.

Migraine headaches come on quite suddenly and recur every few weeks or months. There is almost always pain on only one side of the head, often at the temple. The pain *may* switch sides. The person becomes sensitive to light. Because the victim is nauseated, migraines are sometimes called sick headaches.

Sometimes the person who has a migraine will see spots before the eyes just before it occurs, and some people experience great bursts of energy and activity just prior to the onset of a migraine.

PREVENTION

- If you know your migraine headache comes at a certain time each month, experiment and try to relax and eliminate tension from your life at these times.

HOME TREATMENT

- A mild migraine headache may pass if you go immediately to a darkened room and lie down. Relax the entire body, concentrating on the eyes, the forehead, the jaw and neck muscles, and working down to the toes.
- Most migraine headaches will require professional diagnosis and treatment.

WHEN TO CALL A HEALTH PROFESSIONAL

- If you suspect your headaches are migraine headaches—one-sided, very severe, "sick" headaches. You will need professional diagnosis and evaluation.
- A health professional can provide drugs for treating migraine headaches.
- Discuss with your health professional the new relaxation and "biofeedback" techniques which may prevent migraines.

Headaches in Children

Headaches in children are quite rare but they are more frequent in children whose parents complain of frequent headaches. This is not so much because of inherited physical tendencies but because children are mimics. Therefore, it is wise for parents to mention headaches as infrequently as possible.

Children are susceptible to tension headaches and it is up to a parent to try to discover the cause. Often just talking about a problem may help a child. Some children try to do too much, or are pushed by family or school to do too much. Even "fun" activities can be overdone and the child may be exhausted. Some methods for talking about problems with your children are on page 190.

Hunger can also cause headaches in children. A daily breakfast and a nutritious after-school snack may prevent them. Eyestrain may also cause headaches.

HOME TREATMENT

- Talk to your child and try to discover the source of the headache and eliminate it.
- Play quietly with the child.

- If the headache is still present, have the child lie down in a darkened room with a cool cloth on the forehead. Let the child know you care. "Tension" headaches are sometimes "attention" headaches.
- Aspirin or acetaminophen is rarely needed but, if used, give the correct dose. See page 223 for the proper dosage.

WHEN TO CALL A HEALTH PROFESSIONAL

- If a child's headaches occur 2–3 times a week or more.
- If a headache is severe and is not relieved by relaxation or aspirin.
- If you cannot discover a reasonable cause. Sometimes just talking to a different adult will allow a child to share problems.
- If you suspect eyestrain.

5

Respiratory Problems

Problems in the respiratory system can range from merely bothersome to positively frightening and life-threatening. But whether you have "just" a cold or must deal with a chronic disease, you can learn to manage many ailments in your home and know when professional help is needed.

Whenever anyone complains of an upper respiratory problem, ask first how the person feels. Try to avoid leading questions. If a child complains of a headache, and you ask "Does your throat hurt, too?", you are apt to get an affirmative response. Ask instead "Are you okay, except for the headache?" or "Do you feel bad anywhere else?". Make the patient locate the problem as much as possible.

Then go through the entire home physical exam, starting on page 3. On pages 70–71 is a list of the areas affected by some of the more common upper respiratory complaints. Pay special attention to these areas

in the physical examination. Following each are instructions of "What to Do." If the problem is relatively minor, the appropriate home treatment is suggested. If it is a symptom of more serious disease, then that ailment is referenced. Some topics are quite general and you will be referred to the section covering that topic. Specific symptoms will then be described in that section.

Do not base your action on the first positive symptom you come across. Keep looking and checking off symptoms until you have gone all the way through the chart and reviewed each indicated reference. Strep throat, for example, is often accompanied by white spots on the throat or in the mouth. However, white spots do not necessarily indicate strep throat. They may signal you to look for other symptoms of strep throat. A suspicion of strep throat would then lead you to your physician's office for an exam and a throat culture to verify or disprove it.

Adenoids

The adenoids are lymph tissue located behind the nose. The adenoids become inflamed and swell in upper respiratory infections and may block the eustachian tube, which can lead to middle-ear infections.

The surgical removal of adenoids is called an adenoidectomy. Previously, many children had tonsils and adenoids removed in one operation as a matter of course. Now it is thought that lymph tissue may be helpful in filtering infection and should not be removed without due consideration. It is important to remember that the 2 operations are separate, and each should be considered as a distinct operation.

HOME TREATMENT

Home treatment of adenoid problems should be merely to relieve symptoms before seeing a health professional. Your treatment could include:

- Decongestants which may help nasal stuffiness.
- Small amounts of aspirin for accompanying fever.

WHEN TO CALL A HEALTH PROFESSIONAL

- When a child breathes through the mouth rather than the nose. Discuss this on your next visit to your health professional.
- If there is fever, obstructed nasal breathing, or the nasal and postnasal drainage contains pus.

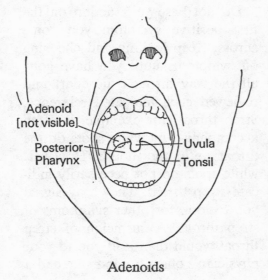

Adenoids

Allergy (Allergic Rhinitis, Hay Fever)

Allergy is the abnormal reaction some people's bodies have to certain substances with which they come in contact.

A person may be allergic to foods or other substances taken by mouth, or things inhaled such as plant pollen or dust. Some people's bodies react to something on the skin or to something injected such as a bee sting or a shot. Allergic reactions range from very mild (itching eyes, sneezing, or runny nose) to very severe (difficulty in breathing, shock, or even circulatory collapse). About 10% of the entire United States population has some kind of allergy at some time during the year.

Allergies appear to be hereditary. Parents with allergies are somewhat more likely to have allergic children. In childhood, allergies differ according to age groups: infants are more likely to be allergic to foods, older children to what they breathe.

The infant who has food allergies is more likely to be allergic to things in the air when older. Suspect allergies if your child has a cold "all winter long" or has a constant runny nose and itchy eyes. The child may rub or pick an itchy nose. The child with allergies may be a mouth-breather at night, snore, and wake with a scratchy sore throat.

Sometimes allergies will be in masquerade. The child may simply be listless and have dark circles under the eyes, or the allergic reaction may be a stomachache or a headache. You need to be a good detective to discover an allergy and its cause. Sometimes even emotional stress can trigger an allergic reaction. Skin rashes and redness are often allergic reactions.

Allergy to substances in the air such as plant pollen can usually be discovered with the use of skin patch tests. Diagnosis for food allergies must be made by trial diets, eliminating and gradually reintroducing suspect foods.

A health professional will usually prescribe antihistamines to relieve the symptoms of allergy while trying to discover the cause.

Once it has been determined that symptoms are indeed caused by allergy, you should weigh the inconvenience of the symptoms against the inconvenience and expense of further treatment. Beyond just giving antihistamines for symptomatic relief, treatment for many allergies includes allergy desensitization shots, which gradually build up resistance to the allergy-causing substances. This treatment, however, is lengthy and expensive. But if the allergy is severe or growing worse, such treatment may indeed be the only solution.

PREVENTION

- If you or your spouse has a history of allergies, consider breast feeding your child. Allergy to breast milk is very rare, but many infants are allergic to cow's milk. Also, there is some evidence that keeping a child on breast milk for 6 months may increase the child's resistance to allergy later. At any rate, by introducing simple solid foods gradually into a diet, any allergy will be more easily found. Milk, wheat, eggs, chocolate, corn, and citrus foods are foods most likely to cause allergic reactions in children. Rice cereal is a

Respiratory Symptom Guide

SYMPTOMS	WHAT TO DO
EYES	

Red, itchy eyes
Matter in eyes
Pussy discharge
	• Think about:
	   ▪ Enough sleep?
	   ▪ Crying?
	   ▪ Windy day?
	• See Allergy, Hayfever, page 68.
	• If accompanied by other symptoms, see Colds, page 78.
	• If unaccompanied by other symptoms, see Conjunctivitis, page 79.
	• If minor, wash with appropriate eye wash.

Runny, tearing eyes	• Note for next health professional visit. • Check for object in eye, see page 137 for removal of object.
Red, burning eyes	• Chance of any chemical in eye? If so, see Chemically Burned Eye, page 130.
NOSE	
Stuffy nose	• See "Your Medicine Chest," page 214.
Nasal discharge — clear (runny nose)	• See Colds, page 78; look for other signs of a cold. • See Allergy, page 68; look for other signs of allergy.

SYMPTOMS	WHAT TO DO
Nasal discharge — green or yellow, thicker discharge	• If unaccompanied by other symptoms, see Object in the Nose, page 137.
Foul nasal odor	• If unaccompanied by other symptoms, see Object in the Nose, page 137.
Nasal Mucosa (tissue in nose)	
Swollen, inflamed	• See Object in the Nose, page 137. Look for other signs of object in nose.
Pale, bluish, boggy	• See Allergy, page 68.
EARS	
	• See Ear Problems, page 84.
FACE	
Pain in face, especially around sinuses	• See Sinusitis, page 94. Look for other symptoms of sinusitis. • See Allergy, page 68 (Sinusitis may occur with allergy.)

SYMPTOMS	WHAT TO DO

MOUTH and THROAT

SYMPTOMS	WHAT TO DO
White spots in mouth or throat	• If unaccompanied by other symptoms, see Canker Sores, page 77. • Also, observe, and if still there in 10 days, call a health professional.
Sores, bleeding in mouth or throat	• If unaccompanied by other symptoms, see Canker Sores, page 77. • May be a sign of dental problems. (Frequent in those with orthodontic appliances.) • If unexplained sores or bleeding continue for more than 5 days, see a health professional.
Bright red patches in throat	• If sore throat is very bright red, see Strep Throat, page 96. • Bright red patches in the throat may be caused by some viral infections, but you should always read the section on Strep Throat when such patches are observed. A health professional must help you distinguish viral from bacterial infections.
Foul odor from mouth, throat	• If accompanied by other symptoms, such as sore throat, see Strep Throat, page 96. • May be a sign of dental problems. • May be a symptom of indigestion. See Indigestion, page 37.
Sore throat	• See Sore Throats, page 95. • See Strep Throat, page 96.

SYMPTOMS	WHAT TO DO
Swollen lymph glands or other lumps on neck	• See Swollen Glands, page 97. • If in adult, or child with no recent disease history, see Mumps, page 92 and Strep Throat, page 96. • If unexplained lumps are seen in throat or mouth or on neck for more than 2 weeks, see a health professional.
Cough	• See Coughs, page 82.

LUNGS

SYMPTOMS	WHAT TO DO
	• See page 22 for how to count respiration.
Wheezing, difficulty in breathing	• See Pneumonia, page 93. • Stop smoking. • See Allergy, page 68. • See Asthma, page 72.
Fast, shallow breathing or difficulty in breathing	• Accompanied by loud cough, see Croup, page 84. • Check for object in mouth, throat. • If severe or prolonged unexplained difficulty in breathing, call health professional.
No respiration	• Perform cardiopulmonary resuscitation (CPR). Get someone else to call health professional. See page 146 for how to perform CPR.

PULSE

SYMPTOMS	WHAT TO DO
	• For how to take pulse, see page 21.
Weak	• See Shock, page 159.

good introduction to solid foods for most children.

- Once the cause of an allergic reaction is found, which may not be at all easy, the best prevention is to avoid that irritant as much as possible.
- Children often outgrow allergies. Thus, you may wish to try to reintroduce foods which cause an infant problems when the child is older.

HOME TREATMENT

- Keep air, especially in sleeping rooms, humidified.
- Keep a diary of all contacts —foods, flowers, weeds, trees, grasses—and relate these to the symptoms.
- Avoid whatever causes allergies. Wear a mask while sweeping a dusty place or cutting grass.
- Keep the home, especially bedrooms, as dust-free as possible. If allergy is severe, you may wish to look into air filters, either portable or those for the whole heating system (precipitron).
- Get extra rest during an allergy attack.
- Oral nasal decongestants or antihistamines may relieve symptoms.
- Blow nose gently to prevent forcing mucus into the

eustachian tube leading from the ear to the throat.
- Stop smoking. The tissues are already irritated.
- House pets should not sleep in or enter the bedroom of the allergic person. In severe cases the pet may have to stay out of the house completely.

WHEN TO CALL A HEALTH PROFESSIONAL

- If allergy causes severe breathing difficulty or wheezing.
- If nasal discharge turns green or yellow.
- If symptoms seem worse over time or inconvenience is great, you and your physician can consider desensitizing shots. These allergy shots help to gradually build immunity to the allergy-causing substance. However, the things you are allergic to may change, or you may move to an area with different irritants.
- A parent can also discuss the possibility of giving allergy shots in the home.

Asthma

Asthma is a severe form of allergic reaction. The bronchial tubes go into spasm and the mucous lining swells, resulting in obstructed breathing. Asthma is the Greek word for panting. The person with an asthmatic attack is literally panting for breath. The person usually coughs a lot and spits up white mucus. The wheeze, a noisy breathing, can be heard some distance away. The person will perspire heavily and the lips and nails may turn bluish. Some asthmatics go into attacks without being exposed to an allergen, but simply from a change in weather or exertion.

Despite these frightening symptoms, asthma is rarely fatal. It can often be prevented using drugs and other methods of treatments, and a severe attack can be relieved by injection.

An asthma attack is a traumatic event. The inability to breathe, even temporarily, produces extreme anxiety in most children and adults. The person's next attack can reactivate the anxiety and even produce more anxiety. This anxiety or panic can be increased if family members become overanxious toward the asthmatic.

PREVENTION

- The best way to prevent asthma is to avoid the irritating substance. However, discovering the irritant is often a difficult task. Sometimes more than one substance is the culprit, and often air pollution, which is difficult to avoid, is a cause. Emotional stress or just worrying about the asthma can trigger an attack.
- Many attacks over a long period of time can lead to emphysema, so every effort should be made to keep asthma under control.
- If the asthmatic starts to become anxious about something, try to calm the person down before an attack occurs.

HOME TREATMENT

- Remain calm when a family member has an attack. Your calmness may reduce the person's anxiety thus lessening the severity of the attack.
- Find and avoid irritating substances as much as possible.
- Try to develop a relaxed mental state.
- Make the bedroom as dust- and irritant-free as possible.
- Consider an air filter (precipitron) which will filter dust particles from the air.
- Get plenty of rest and exercise. Rest allows your body's energy to fight the disease and exercise will help strengthen the lungs.
- Get extra fluids to thin bronchial mucus.
- Stop smoking and avoid people who are smoking.

WHEN TO CALL A HEALTH PROFESSIONAL

- Anyone who is subject to acute allergy attacks should discuss with his or her health professional exactly what should be done when an attack begins. Once asthma patients develop a good understanding of and confidence in their asthma medications, they can handle most acute attacks without immediate professional help.
- To discuss allergy desensitization shots, which may be useful in preventing asthma.
- If sputum is green, yellow, or bloody. This may be a sign of a secondary bacterial infection.
- If the victim and family members become more and more anxious with each attack, it may be helpful to see a health professional. The family could learn to deal realistically with the asthmatic and not reject or over-protect the victim.
- If the asthmatic is over-anxious, relief can sometimes be found by meeting with other asthmatics who have dealt successfully with attacks. One way to do this is to inform your health professional that you would like to talk with another parent who has an asthmatic child. Your health professional can contact such parents and give them your name and telephone number. Use of this method will insure that there is no lack of confidentiality.

Bacterial Infections

Generally, a bacterial infection is more serious than a viral infection. Complications such as kidney and heart problems can set in. Therefore, it is necessary that a bacterial infection be treated promptly.

Bacteria-caused upper respiratory infections are often hard to distinguish from those which are caused by a virus. Often the only way they can be discovered is by culturing them in a laboratory. A tissue scraping or a bit of exudate (mucus, pus, or phlegm) is placed on a growth plate and "grown out." The growth can then be analyzed and identified if it is a bacteria. This process takes about 24–48 hours.

Most bacteria-caused infections are cured fairly easily with antibiotic drugs, but it is important that not all infections be treated as bacterial infections. There are good and bad bacteria. Antibiotics destroy both types and thus should be used only when necessary. Sometimes women who have been treated for a bacterial infection come down with a urinary tract infection. That's because the "good" bacteria in the urinary tract were eliminated by the antibiotic treatment. The organisms (often yeast) which those bacteria controlled could then grow quickly.

Another reason to use antibiotics only when necessary is that bacteria subjected to antibiotics can build up resistant strains—the strong survive, making later treatment more difficult. It's also possible for a person to develop an allergy to an antibiotic, so that it cannot be used when really needed.

Often bacteria will attack the already weakened system of a person with a viral infection. Thus bacterial infections sometimes follow viral infections, particularly if the viral infection is not given proper home treatment.

The most common bacterial complications of viral upper respiratory infections are ear infections and strep throat (streptococcus bacteria). Impetigo is another strep infection and it will need professional help if at all extensive. *You cannot prevent complications of a viral infection by starting antibiotic therapy.* Once a bacterial infection is suspected, there is usually time to verify it and treat it without endangering the patient. Therefore, it is important to remember that only one-tenth of all infections will respond to antibiotic treatment; *you should not expect your health professional to prescribe an antibiotic treatment before seeing the patient,* and if necessary, taking a culture to verify presence of a bacterial infection.

WHEN TO CALL A HEALTH PROFESSIONAL

- If there is a high fever (over 103°) accompanying any illness.
- If the person is not starting to improve after 4 days.
- If sputum or nasal discharge turns from white or clear to yellow or green or is bloody.
- If a cough lingers after a cold for more than 5 days without improvement. You may have a non-productive cough 7–9 days after a cold. If other symptoms are clearing, there's no need to see a health professional.

Bronchitis

Bronchitis is an inflammation of the lower windpipe and the bronchial tubes which carry air to and from the lungs. In bronchitis the bronchial tubes are injured by the infection and secrete a sticky mucus. It becomes increasingly difficult for the cilia or hairs on the bronchi to clean out this mucus.

Bronchitis often occurs after a cold or upper respiratory infection which doesn't cure completely. It may be caused by a virus or a bacterium and is much more common among smokers or those who work in polluted air. *Seventy-five percent of patients with chronic bronchitis have a history of heavy smoking.*

The body attempts to clear out the sticky mucus through the cough, the most significant symptom of bronchitis. Other symptoms are tiredness, low fever, sore throat, runny nose, and sometimes, wheezing. The treatment for bronchitis is basically to help that cough clear out the mucus.

Untreated bronchitis can lead to pneumonia. Chronic bronchitis can lead to chronic obstructive pulmonary disease (emphysema), a very serious, incurable ailment.

PREVENTION

Give proper home care to minor respiratory problems such as colds. Stopping smoking during a cold may help prevent the irritation to the cilia and decrease the chance of complications.

HOME TREATMENT

- Drink a large amount of fluids—as much as a gallon a day. Liquids help thin the mucus in the lungs, making it easier to clean out. This is the most important part of treatment.
- Rest in bed. The lungs need lots of rest to cure themselves.
- Stop smoking—it irritates the tissue and slows healing.
- Inhale steam frequently from a vaporizer or over the bathroom sink. Steam inhalation will dilute mucus and help the cough bring it up.
- Take expectorant cough medicines to help bring up the mucus. See "Your Medicine Chest," page 225, for examples of cough medicines.
- Twice daily, lie on your stomach and hang your head and chest over the side of the bed for one minute. This procedure, called postural drainage, helps drain the mucus. Any of several methods which get the head lower than the chest will work.
- Massage the chest and back muscles. Use Vicks Vaporub, Ben Gay, or a similar over-the-counter preparation, if desired. The massaging increases blood flow to the chest and aids relaxation.

WHEN TO CALL A HEALTH PROFESSIONAL

- If sputum, usually clear or white, is green, brown, or yellow. This can indicate bacterial infection and requires antibiotic treatment.
- If the mucus coughed up becomes thick and "rusty" colored.
- If there is a history of frequent bronchitis.
- If breathing difficulty is

present when not coughing.
- If there is wheezing.
- If there is increasing chest pain.
- If mucus continues to thicken.
- If patient is an infant, elderly, or chronically ill.

- If a sore is very painful or comes back frequently.
- If white spots that are not canker sores appear in the mouth and do not heal within 10 days.

Canker Sores

Canker sores are little blisters on the membranes of the mouth and cheek which break and leave open sores. These sores usually heal by themselves in about 10 days, but they can be very painful.

No one knows for sure what causes canker sores, but some people are more susceptible than others.

HOME TREATMENT

- Avoid eating spicy or salty foods, or citrus fruits when you have a canker sore.
- Apply an oral paste, like Orabase, to the canker sore. It sticks to the sore and protects it, eases the pain and speeds healing.
- Baking soda and water mixed to a thin paste may bring relief.

WHEN TO SEE A HEALTH PROFESSIONAL

- If a canker sore, or any sore, does not heal within 10–14 days.

Cold Sores

Cold sores or fever blisters, caused by a Herpes virus, are small red blisters which often weep and scab and have a dry ring around a moist center. Canker sores appear inside the mouth, while cold sores are outside the mouth. Cold sores are sometimes confused with impetigo, but while impetigo is usually between the nose and upper lip, cold sores usually appear on the lower lip or the outer edge of the mouth. The fluid from impetigo is pussy but the fluids in cold sores are clear. Cold sores may appear after colds, with a fever, after exposure to the sun, associated with menstruation, or for no apparent reason at all.

HOME TREATMENT

- Be patient. Cold sores usually go away within 7–10 days.
- Chapstick, Blistex, or another lip balm may ease the pain.
- Cornstarch may be soothing. Apply in a paste made with a little water.

Colds (Viral Rhinitis, Pharyngitis)

The common cold is an inflammation of the membranes of the nose, throat, pharynx, or tonsils. Infection can spread to the bronchi and middle ear. A cold is always virus-caused and there is no immunization. A cold cannot be cured by antibiotics, but occasionally the complications of a cold may be treated with an antibiotic. Antibiotics *do not* prevent complications.

Colds occur throughout the year, but are most common in late winter and early spring. The average child has 6 colds a year, adults much fewer.

The symptoms of a cold are runny nose, red, itchy eyes, sneezing, sore throat, coughing, headache, and general body aches. As a cold progresses, nasal mucus may become superficially contaminated with bacteria and become pussy and thick. This is the stage just before a cold dries up. Children often have a fever with a cold, but fever in adults with a cold is less common. A cold usually lasts 2 weeks in a child and should be gone in a week in an adult. There is a gradual 1 or 2 day onset.

Frequently a cold will lead to more serious complications. These are sometimes caused by improper or no home treatment, but some people, especially children, are more susceptible to complications. Ear infections, tonsillitis, and strep throat are 3 such complications.

You should be able to recognize symptoms that warn of these.

You should suspect strep throat and go to your health professional for a culture if, during a cold: the throat becomes very sore and/or bright red or spotty, the clear nasal discharge turns green or yellow, there is an overall foul odor from the mouth or throat, or a fever of 103° is present. An earache, which is more than just a feeling of fullness in the ear following a cold, should also be investigated by your health professional.

If it seems you or your child has a cold all the time, or if cold symptoms last 3 weeks or more, suspect allergy. See page 68 for symptoms of allergy.

PREVENTION

Colds are almost an inevitable fact of life, but there are some hints which might help you prevent a cold, especially during the "cold" months of late winter and early spring.

- Eat and sleep properly and get plenty of exercise to keep up your resistance.
- Wash your hands frequently, particularly when you're around people with colds.
- Keep your hands away from your nose, eyes, and mouth.
- Humidify at least the bedroom.

- Using mouthwash won't prevent a cold.

HOME TREATMENT

- Get extra rest after work or school. The person with a cold needs extra rest, but it is not necessary to stay home from work or school if you feel well enough to accomplish something, providing you don't needlessly expose others.
- Drink extra fluids. Double or triple your normal fluid intake.
- Take aspirin or acetaminophen (Tylenol, Nebs, Datril) to reduce fever and relieve aches and pain. See dosage chart, page 223.
- Humidify the patient's bedroom for comfort.
- Some over-the-counter preparations *may* relieve the symptoms of a cold, making the patient more comfortable. They will not shorten the length of a cold. Decongestants, antihistamines, cough syrups, cough drops, or nose drops may be helpful. Their purpose and use is explained in "Your Medicine Chest," page 223. Sometimes use of decongestants at the first sign of a cold may prevent onset of an ear infection.

- Antibiotics will not help a cold.

WHEN TO CALL A HEALTH PROFESSIONAL

- Fever over 103° with other symptoms of a cold.
- Wheezing or breathing difficulty.
- A very sore, bright red, or spotty throat.
- An overall foul odor from the throat, nose, or ears.
- A yellow or green nasal discharge rather than clear.
- Cough which persists more than 5 days after a cold without improving.
- Earache lasting more than an hour, more than just "stuffy."
- If the patient does not seem to be improving or if you are quite concerned.

Conjunctivitis

Conjunctivitis, or pinkeye, can be caused by bacteria, a virus, or by irritation from polluted air. It usually will clear by itself, or your health professional can prescribe some antibiotic eye drops. The symptoms of pinkeye are redness in the whites of the eyes or excess matter in the eyes, without other upper respiratory symptoms. Some redness or swelling of the eyes is quite common with many respiratory infections and allergies and is not serious. With conjunctivitis, the lower lid will be red and swollen on the inside. The person may complain of a sandy, scratchy feeling in the eyes.

PREVENTION

Because conjunctivitis is very contagious, it is important for you to wash your hands thoroughly after treating a person with pinkeye. Just by rubbing the eyes, a child can transfer the condition from one eye to the other, so try to keep your child from eye rubbing. Hands should be washed often. Conjunctivitis can spread to the whole family quite quickly.

HOME TREATMENT

- Prevent spreading of the disease.
- Sometimes pus or matter in the eye will cake and dry during the night and on waking the person is unable to open the eyes. Lightly wipe the eyes with moist cotton or a clean washcloth and water.
- Do not cover the eye with a patch.
- If eye drops are prescribed, insert in the following manner: pull the lower lid down with 2 fingers making a little pouch and put the drops in there. Close the eye to let the drop move around. Be sure the

dropper is clean and does not touch any surface. Eye drops are washed out by normal tearing in about 20 minutes, so they should be replaced about once an hour.

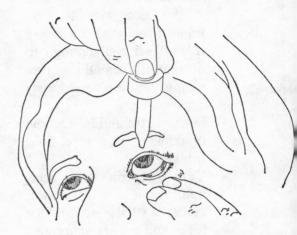

Inserting eye drops

WHEN TO CALL A HEALTH PROFESSIONAL

- If eye is red with thick, pussy discharge.
- If the problem is very bothersome or recurring, a health professional can prescribe eye drops.
- If there is distinct pain in the eye rather than irritation.
- If there is an abnormal difference in size of pupils. A constricted pupil may indicate iritis, which needs professional treatment.

Convulsion—Febrile (With Fever) in Children

Convulsions or fits are involuntary spasms of muscles which may involve the whole body or only part of it. Although frightening, convulsions in children between 6 months and 4 years of age usually do *not* indicate any serious ailment.

Convulsions are more likely to occur when children have a high fever. Some young children's temperature-regulating mechanisms are not completely developed, and their bodies can't perspire enough to cool the body quickly.

The child with a convulsion stiffens up, clenching fists and teeth. The eyes will roll back and the child will hold his or her breath, salivate a lot and maybe turn a little blue. Often the child will lose urine or pass stools.

PREVENTION

- Dress a child with a fever loosely to prevent overheating.
- If your child has a tendency to convulsions, discuss with your health professional the possibility of fever-reducing suppositories which prevent convulsions if given at the onset of a fever.
- Much depends on how sick the child appears. A fever is a sign that the body is fighting infection. There is usually no need to reduce a fever under 101° (102° rectally).
- As fever climbs, observe the child. A fever of 103° in a child who otherwise looks okay need not be reduced. But if the fever goes over 103°, to 104° or higher, it should be reduced.
- Most convulsions occur with fevers of 105° or higher.
- Children run much higher fevers than adults. A fever of 103–104° is considered quite high in an adult.

HOME TREATMENT

- Protect the child from falling against a table edge or some other sharp object.
- Time the length of the convulsion, if possible.
- Roll the child to the side to drain saliva from the mouth. Clear mouth of any vomit or saliva so the child can breathe.
- There is not much point in trying to put a blunt object between the teeth; either you'll break the stick or a few teeth.
- To reduce fever, sponge the child with cool (not cold) cloths or immerse in lukewarm water. Some shivering indicates the child is cooling rapidly.
- Do not use ice packs. That

82

is too sudden a reduction.

- Check for injuries.
- Dress the child lightly, and put her or him to sleep in a cool room.
- Try to stay calm. This will greatly help the child.
- After the convulsion is over, encourage the child to take extra fluids.

WHEN TO CALL A HEALTH PROFESSIONAL

- If the convulsion is not accompanied by fever.
- If it is the child's first convulsion.
- If the child is under 6 months old or is 5 years or older or if convulsion is in adult.
- If the convulsion lasts longer than 1 minute.
- If you are unable to successfully reduce the fever after a convulsion. You should reduce it to 101° to be sure it is well below the seizure-producing level.

Coughs

Coughing is the way the body expels foreign bodies and mucus from the lower respiratory tract. While a cough's loudness only shows the degree of effort put into the cough, all coughs have distinct characteristics you can learn to recognize. A dry, hacking cough indicates something is irritating the respiratory tract. Loose and juicy coughs indicate mucus is being produced. This mucus often flips over the esophagus and gets swallowed, and then appears in the vomit or stool.

There are 3 types of coughs. The productive cough is one that produces phlegm or mucus which comes up with coughing. The nonproductive cough is a dry cough, producing no mucus. A reflex cough is one that is a result of a disturbance or irritation which may or may not be associated with the respiratory tract; it may originate in the vocal cords, the ear, or even the stomach.

In general, the simplest cure for any cough is water. Water helps to loosen phlegm and soothe an irritated throat. Dry, hacking coughs often respond to honey in hot water, tea, or lemon juice. Suppressants to control the cough and expectorants which liquify the mucus and make it easier to bring up are 2 drugs that may help. Detailed descriptions of these drugs can be found on page 225. Cough drops can soothe the irritated parts of your mouth and accessible parts of your throat, but they have no effect on the cough-producing mechanism. They reduce the tickling irritation in the back of your throat. Expensive medicinally flavored cough drops are not any better than the inexpensive candy-flavored ones or plain old hard candy.

Description and Treatment of Coughs

DESCRIPTION OF COUGH	POSSIBLE CAUSE	HOME TREATMENT
Seal-like bark	Croup	See page 84.
Wheezing, noisy breathing out	Allergy Asthma	See page 68. See page 72.
Dry coughs that occur only in the morning and seem better after breakfast	Dry air	Increase fluids. Use a humidifier in the bedroom. See page 211.
	Cigarettes	
Hacking, dry, non-productive coughs	Postnasal drip	Increase fluids. Decongestants are helpful.
	Cigarettes	
A dry, sudden onset cough that appears immediately following a choking episode, most often in a large infant or toddler	Foreign Object	See page 150 for how to remove the object.
Dry coughs occurring intermittently day and night especially with a fever	Respiratory infection	Increase fluids. Use a suppressant at night and expectorants during the day.
Chronic cough following a cold	Bronchitis	See page 75.

WHEN TO CALL A HEALTH PROFESSIONAL

- If the non-productive cough suddenly becomes productive.
- If mucus becomes thick or green.
- If there is blood in the sputum on several occasions.
- If the cough lasts more than 5 days without improvement.
- If the cough suddenly gets worse.
- If the cough is accompanied by a fever of 103°.

Croup

Croup is a respiratory problem of children 2–4 years of age. It usually occurs around midnight in the winter time. A child with croup has a hacking cough, a seal-like bark, and has trouble breathing. The child is terrified and fighting for breath with a low-grade fever of 100–101°.

HOME TREATMENT

- Stay calm. The child is already terrified and needs you to be calm.
- Get moisture into the air to make it easier for the child to breathe. The simplest method is to take the child into the bathroom, turn on all the hot water faucets, then both of you sit on the floor and read a story in the steamy room.
- Set up a vaporizer or croup tent in the child's bedroom. Another member of the family could do this while you are still in the bathroom with the child. To make a croup tent, put a humidifier under the crib and drape a blanket over the head of the crib to trap the moisture near the child's head. If the child is older and no longer in a crib, you can drape the blanket over an umbrella or card table. With a cold mist humidifier, the air will be quite cold but you need

not worry about your child getting too chilled. The humidity is the important part.
- If the child starts crying, the worst is over. Someone who can cry can breathe.

WHEN TO CALL A HEALTH PROFESSIONAL

- If croup lasts longer than 3 nights.
- If 20 minutes of steam inhalation does not relax the child enough to allow sleep.
- If the child is gasping and can't breathe.
- If there is a "sucking-in," or retraction between the ribs as the child breathes in.
- If the child has a high fever of 102–103°.
- If you or your child becomes hysterical and cannot seem to calm down.
- If it is the first case of croup in your family.
- A very late sign to call your health professional is if the child's skin turns bluish or dusky. This is a sign that the child is not getting enough oxygen and is very serious.

Ear Problems

Ears are subject to a variety of problems. The symptoms and suggestion of what to do on page 86

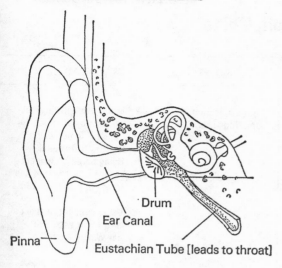

Pinna

Drum

Ear Canal

Eustachian Tube [leads to throat]

Ear

will direct you to the appropriate section of Ear Problems.

Ear Wax

The production of ear wax is perfectly normal. It is a protective secretion, similar to mucus or tears, which filters dust and keeps the ear clean. Normally ear wax is liquid, self-draining, and not a cause for concern. Occasionally, however, the wax will build up, become crusty, turn black, and cause some hearing loss. Poking at the wax with cotton swabs, fingers, or other devices will only further compact the wax against the eardrum. Although professional help using specialized tools is needed to remove tightly packed wax, you can handle most ear wax problems by avoiding cotton swabs and following the home treatment tips below.

Children have a lot of ear wax. It seems to taper off as they grow older. You should be concerned only if the ear wax causes ringing or a "full" feeling in the ears, or some hearing loss.

HOME TREATMENT

- Lie down with a warm cloth under the affected ear. This should cause the wax to soften and drain out.
- Stand under a warm shower with waxy ear tilted toward showerhead. The warm water should help loosen the wax.
- If the warm cloth and shower do not work, apply Debrox, Cerumenex, or some other over-the-counter wax softener each night for 3–4 days. Put in 5 drops at bedtime and apply a hot water bottle or heating pad set at medium heat to the ear for 15 minutes. Tilt the head so the ear is over a handkerchief or tissue and gently remove excess solution.

WHEN TO CALL A HEALTH PROFESSIONAL

- If above procedures do not work. If wax build-up is hard, dry, and impacted, it may take up to 3 visits to remove it.

Ear Symptom Guide

SYMPTOMS	WHAT TO DO
EAR PROBLEMS	
Pain in ear	• See Middle Ear Infections, page 86.
Outer ear tender, painful when wiggled	• See Swimmer's Ear, page 88. • If preceded by a cold, see Middle Ear Infections, page 86.
Crusty, pussy discharge	• See Swimmer's Ear, page 88. • If preceded by earache and then pain subsides after you notice discharge, see Middle Ear Infection, page 86.
Fullness, feeling of something in ear	• See Swimmer's Ear, page 88. • If accompanied by other symptoms, see Colds, page 78.

SYMPTOMS	WHAT TO DO
Fullness, feeling of something in ear	• Using penlight, inspect ear for object in ear. If object is in ear, call a health professional. • Using penlight, inspect ear for insect in ear. See Insect in Ear, page 135. • Using penlight, inspect ear for ear wax. See Ear Wax, page 85.
Itching, burning in ear	• See Swimmer's Ear, page 88.
Hearing loss, nonattentiveness	• See Ear Wax, page 85. • If continues over 10 days, see a health professional.
Pulling at ears by infants, small children	• See Middle Ear Infections, page 86.

Middle Ear Infections (Otitis Media)

Middle ear infections are almost always bacterially caused. The viral infection of a cold causes tissue in the eustachian tube to swell. The eustachian tube carries air from ear to throat, and equalizes pressure between the middle ear and the outside world. As the tube is gradually closed off, a vacuum is created and fluids seep in, providing an excellent breeding ground for bacteria. White cells and body fluids come to fight the infection, causing pressure on the eardrum and pain. Sometimes the pressure builds to a point where the eardrum ruptures and the fluid leaks out, thus equalizing the pressure. While this is nature's way of healing and is not necessarily harmful, repeated ruptures of the drum can cause scarring and possible hearing loss.

Left untreated, the bacteria can spread to the skull bones or brain. Fortunately, antibiotics will control the growth of bacteria and prevent such complications.

When an ear infection sets in, professional help is needed.

Ear infections are more common in young children because their eustachian tubes are narrow and block more easily. Also, they have more colds. It has been found that parents who had frequent childhood earaches often have children with earaches, indicating that anatomy apparently plays a role. Ear infections can also be caused by careless, hard blowing of the nose or by excessive sniffing which sends bacteria up the eustachian tube.

Because small children cannot tell you it hurts, the first sign of an earache might be a pulling or tugging on the ears. It is important to notice, because untreated ear infections can readily cause hearing loss in children under 3.

Serous otitis media is a non-bacterial, less painful ear infection. Usually the only symptoms are temporary hearing loss or temporary fullness in the ear. If only these symptoms are present, there is no need to see a health professional, unless they continue more than 10 days.

Symptoms of a bacterial ear infection or earache will be pain, dizziness, ringing or fullness in ears, hearing loss, fever, headache, and runny nose.

PREVENTION

Blow your nose gently. Treat a cold rapidly, especially if you are susceptible to ear infections. In some cases, oral decongestants taken at the onset of a cold will prevent eustachian tube blockage and thus prevent an ear infection.

HOME TREATMENT

After calling a health professional, the following may help relieve pain:

- Heat applied to the ear will ease the pain. Use a warm washcloth or a heating pad.
- If the pain is severe, use ear drops to relieve the ache until a health professional is available. The drops will not reduce the need for antibiotic treatment, but will usually allow you to wait until morning to see a health professional.
- Rest. Let your energy go to fighting the infection.
- Oral nasal decongestants may help relieve earache.
- Aspirin or acetaminophen will help relieve the pain of earache.

WHEN TO CALL A HEALTH PROFESSIONAL

- Any earache that lasts over 1 hour and is accompanied by acute pain should be checked by a health professional within 24 hours of the first pain. If the pain is severe at night, call the next morning *even if the pain has stopped*. The infection may still be present even if pain has subsided and should at least be discussed with a health professional.
- Take the full course of anti-

biotic, if prescribed, but call if there is any adverse reaction to the antibiotic and stop taking it.

- If pain increases despite treatment.
- If temperature is over 102°.
- If patient cannot touch chin to chest without pain. This may be a sign of meningitis.
- If a rupture is suspected.

Swimmer's Ear (Otitis Externa)

Swimmer's ear is an infection of the external ear canal. It is called swimmer's ear because it often appears after one has been swimming or otherwise has gotten the ear filled with water.

The first symptom of swimmer's ear is a feeling of tenderness or fullness in the ear, as if water were in it. The person may complain of itching and burning in the ears, and wiggling the outer ear will cause pain.

More acute swimmer's ear will cause redness of the ear canal and a crusty, pussy discharge. These acute symptoms indicate a secondary bacterial infection has set in, and this more acute secondary infection must be treated.

PREVENTION

Drying the ear carefully immediately after swimming may control swimmer's ear. One simple, safe method: twist each of the 4 corners of a facial tissue into a tip. With head tipped to the left, gently place the tissue tip into the left ear canal. Each of the 4 corners should be held in place for a count of 10. Dry the right ear with the 4 corners of a second facial tissue.

Swim teams have found that recurring swimmer's ear can also be prevented by using prescription ear drops which change the acid/alkali level in the ear canal.

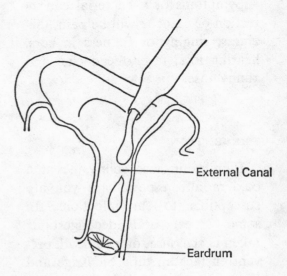

External Canal

Eardrum

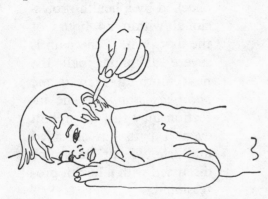

Inserting ear drops

HOME TREATMENT

- Look in the ear with a penlight to be sure there is not an object or an insect in the ear. See Insect in the Ear, page 135.
- If drops are prescribed, you need to know how to insert them. Have the person lie down, ear facing up. You may find it easier to insert ear drops in a small child in the following manner: Hold the child on your lap with legs around your waist and head down between your legs. Place drops on the canal wall in small quantities, so air can escape up the other side. If air gets trapped under the drops, it will keep the solution from penetrating any further. If drops don't go down, try to wiggle the ear to get them down where they will be effective.

WHEN TO CALL A HEALTH PROFESSIONAL

- For antifungal drops which may cure swimmer's ear. However, it will probably recur.
- For ear drops which change acid/alkali level, and may prevent the problem.
- If there is a bloody or pussy discharge.
- If the earache follows a cold.

Emphysema (Chronic Obstructive Pulmonary Disease)

Emphysema is a chronic lung condition caused by repeated irritation or infection of the tissues of the lungs. Over the years, repeated irritation by cigarette smoke, pollution, or infection stretches the elastic lung tissue so it cannot expand and contract properly. Emphysema is much more likely to occur in the person who has been a heavy cigarette smoker for a long time. The lungs lose their ability to add oxygen to the blood and the person is susceptible to frequent attacks of bronchitis. Symptoms of emphysema are shortness of breath on exertion, frequent respiratory infections and bronchitis, wheezing, and chronic cough.

PREVENTION

Emphysema is caused by irritants to the lungs. Therefore, elimination of as many of those irritants as possible can help to prevent emphysema. Avoid pollution, and if you work where the air is polluted, do what you can to filter the air and control dust and irritants. You should also know that cigarette smoking is a known contributor to emphysema.

HOME TREATMENT

Emphysema must be diagnosed by a health professional. Once diagnosed, a detailed routine will be prescribed. There is no cure for emphysema, but proper treatment can help you lead a more normal life. Be sure you understand all instructions for the control of your disease.

WHEN TO CALL A HEALTH PROFESSIONAL

- If you have shortness of breath on exertion.
- If you have frequent respiratory infections, especially bronchitis.
- If you have a chronic cough.
- If you have persistent wheezing.
- If you are a heavy smoker and want help quitting.

Encephalitis

Encephalitis is an inflammation of the brain, generally caused by a viral or bacterial infection. Mild encephalitis may occur with many diseases, even mumps or chicken pox.

The most common symptoms of encephalitis are high fever, headache, nausea, vomiting, and excessive sleepiness.

WHEN TO CALL A HEALTH PROFESSIONAL

- If any of the above symptoms—high fever (103°), severe headache, nausea, vomiting, or excessive

sleepiness—accompany or follow a viral or bacterial illness.
- If any of the above symptoms occur following a mosquito bite. In some states, equine encephalitis is transmitted by mosquitoes.

Influenza

Influenza, often called flu, is a viral illness which occurs commonly in the winter. It usually appears in epidemic form and affects many members of a community. Influenza has symptoms similar to a cold, but they are usually more severe and come on quite suddenly.

The most characteristic symptoms of influenza are weakness and fatigue. Others are muscle aches, headaches, fever (101–102°), sneezes, and a runny nose.

Although a person feels very sick with influenza, it rarely leads to more serious complications. The disease is usually dangerous only for infants, the elderly, or the chronically ill.

PREVENTION

Immunization against influenza provides fair protection, or may lessen symptoms if the disease is contracted. The elderly or chronically ill should be immunized. The immunization is given each fall in anticipation of the coming flu season. You must be immunized within 1 week to 4 months prior to exposure for the shots to be effective.

HOME TREATMENT

- Bed rest will be needed.
- Drink extra fluids, at least 1 full glass every hour.
- Aspirin or acetaminophen can relieve head and muscle aches. See dosage chart, page 223.
- Antihistamines may help dry up mucus, help the patient breathe more easily, and feel more comfortable.

WHEN TO CALL A HEALTH PROFESSIONAL

- If cough brings up heavy mucus.
- After 5 days of fever over 102°.
- If there is increasing difficulty in breathing.
- When a patient seemingly gets better, then gets worse again.

Laryngitis & Hoarseness

Laryngitis is a viral or bacterial infection of the voice box or larynx. The most common cause is a cold but it can also be produced by allergy. Hoarseness can be caused by yelling or cigarette smoke and displays similar symptoms.

Symptoms of laryngitis are an urge to clear your throat, fever, tiredness, pain in throat, coughing, and loss of voice.

PREVENTION

- If you have a respiratory infection, take time to treat it so that the infection won't spread to your voice box.
- To prevent hoarseness, stop shouting as soon as you feel minor pain. Give your vocal cords a rest.

HOME TREATMENT

- It will usually heal itself in 5–10 days and medication will do little to speed recovery.
- If it is caused by a cold, treat the cold. See page 78.
- Rest your voice by not shouting and by talking little.
- Stop smoking and avoid other people's smoke.
- Humidify the air.
- Drink lots of liquids.
- To soothe the throat gargle with warm salt water (1 tsp. in 8 oz. of water) or drink honey in hot water, lemon juice, or weak tea.

WHEN TO CALL A HEALTH PROFESSIONAL

- If you suspect a bacterial infection (see page 74).

• If hoarseness isn't associated with a viral infection or smoking, and persists for 1 month.

sterile if they get the mumps. Females won't become sterile, but mumps can go to the ovaries which can be very painful.

Mumps

Mumps, once a common childhood illness, is another disease being conquered through immunization. When a person gets mumps, the parotid gland, located in front of and below the earlobe, swells on one or both sides. To help determine if it is mumps, run your finger down the jawline. If it is mumps the jawbone will not be felt. If it is swollen lymph glands the jawbone can still be felt. This swelling may be accompanied by fever and vomiting. The person is contagious from 1 day before the swelling begins until the swelling has gone down, at least 7 days.

Mumps can *occasionally* lead to encephalitis, an inflammation of the brain, to deafness, or to sterility in males after puberty.

PREVENTION

Your child should be immunized after 12 months of age. There is now a convenient measles-mumps-rubella shot for children which can be given all at once. Only 1 shot is necessary for life-long immunity. Adults who have never had mumps should be immunized against them. Males, after puberty, can become

HOME TREATMENT

• Give extra fluids. It may be more comfortable for the patient to sip through a straw.
• Isolate the patient until the swelling subsides.
• Sucking ice may ease vomiting.

WHEN TO CALL A HEALTH PROFESSIONAL

• If the fever goes over 103°.
• If the patient has a severe headache.

Object in the Nose

Quite often curious children will put something such as a bead or a piece of popcorn up their noses. With a little patience, you often can save a physician visit by removing a foreign object yourself.

If the child does not tell you right away what has happened, you'll get some clues in a few days. A very foul-smelling green or yellow discharge from just 1 nostril is a strong hint that there is an object in the nose. The mucous membranes are also swollen, and there may be tenderness in the nose.

HOME TREATMENT

- Spray a nasal decongestant in the affected nostril. (See "Your Medicine Chest," page 223.) This will reduce the swelling of the membranes, and sometimes the object will drop out.
- Using a good light and holding the child quiet, try to remove the foreign object with blunt-nose tweezers. If you do not succeed after 2 tries, call a health professional.
- The nostril may bleed a little. This is not serious.

Pneumonia

Pneumonia is an infection of the smallest air passages (the alveoli) in your lungs. It can be caused by a variety of bacteria or viruses. Pneumonia often follows another upper respiratory illness, especially in elderly people or in people whose resistance is poor due to inadequate diet, overexposure to the cold, or fatigue. While cold air cannot of itself *cause* illness, it can lower your body's resistance. Improper home treatment of a minor upper respiratory illness may lead to pneumonia.

Usually the person with pneumonia will appear very ill. The first signal of the disease, especially in a child, is very rapid breathing. An older person may have pain in the chest, especially when coughing or taking a deep breath, and may cough up green or brown sputum. This is mucus from deep in the lung. Each breath is labored. There are often shaking chills and fever.

PREVENTION

The most important aspect of preventing pneumonia is adequate care of minor illnesses. Keeping up the body's normal resistance with adequate diet, rest, and exercise may help prevent pneumonia from developing.

HOME TREATMENT

A health professional must be called if you suspect pneumonia. After a diagnosis of pneumonia, follow the home treatment below.

- Pneumonia requires lots of rest for the lungs to clear themselves.
- Extra fluids are necessary to help thin mucus. Give adults and children at least an 8 ounce glass every hour.

WHEN TO CALL A HEALTH PROFESSIONAL

- If during any respiratory illness, there is rapid or labored breathing.
- If a cough following a cold lasts longer than 5 days without improving.
- If an unexplained cough appears a few weeks after a cold.

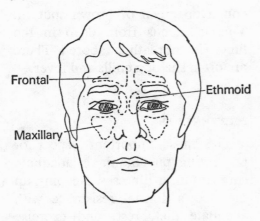

Frontal

Ethmoid

Maxillary

Sinus cavities

Sinusitis

Sinusitis is an inflammation of the sinuses. The sinuses are cavities lined with mucous membranes, which drain easily unless there is an infection. There are 2 categories of sinus infections: acute, lasting less than 3 weeks, and chronic, lasting longer. Because the sinus cavities are not completely developed until late adolescence, sinus infections are seldom found in young children.

The key symptom to sinus infection is pain in the face under the eyes and opposite the bridge of the nose. There may also be headache, fever, runny nose, postnasal drip (mucus running down the throat), sore throat, and toothaches. Headaches may occur on rising and get worse in the afternoon.

To distinguish sinus pain from toothache, jump up and down on your heels. If the pain is from a sinus infection, it will be felt above the teeth. If a toothache is causing the pain, it will center on the tooth.

PREVENTION

Improper, too forceful blowing of the nose can cause sinus infections by forcing mucus up into a sinus and blocking it. Prompt, correct treatment of a cold may prevent a sinus infection.

HOME TREATMENT

- When you first notice sinus pain, lie down on your back and apply alternating hot and cold compresses to your forehead and cheeks, about 1 minute each, for 10 minutes. If needed, repeat 4 times daily, giving the last treatment at bedtime. This treatment seems to stimulate the flow of mucus.
- Apply decongestant nose drops to each nostril while lying down. See page 223 for types of decongestants. Try repeating the letter K (kay-kay-kay) for 30 seconds. This can help open the sinuses.
- Gargle with warm water to clear the throat of draining mucus.
- Increase home humidity, especially bedrooms.
- Drink extra fluids to keep mucus thin. Drink 3 times your normal intake.
- Breathe steam from a vaporizer or over a sink filled with hot water.
- You may take aspirin or

acetaminophen for headache. See page 223 for dosage.

WHEN TO CALL A HEALTH PROFESSIONAL

- If you feel pain along the ridge between the nose and lower eyelid. This could indicate infection of the ethmoid sinus, which is quite serious. Before the era of antibiotics this complication often led to meningitis and death.
- Fever over 101°.
- Increased swelling of the face.
- Severe headache not eased by aspirin or acetaminophen.
- Bleeding from the nose.
- Increased thick yellow or green nasal discharge.
- Changes or blurring in vision.
- No improvement after 2 days of home treatment.

Sore Throats (Mild)

You should usually be able to trace the cause of a mild sore throat. Often a mild sore throat is due to low humidity, smoking, air pollution, perhaps yelling. People with allergies and stuffy noses may breathe through their mouths while sleeping, thus causing a mild sore throat on rising. Sometimes a mild sore throat accompanies a cold.

PREVENTION

An irritated throat may be prevented by avoiding the irritant. For example, try increasing the humidity of your living and working environments.

HOME TREATMENT

- Humidify the home, especially the bedroom.
- A mild sore throat can be eased by gargling with hot salt water (1 tsp. in 8 oz. water), or with Cepacol or another commercial mouthwash.
- Sucking cough drops or hard candy may soothe irritated tissue.
- Honey and lemon or weak tea may help.
- Drinking more fluids will soothe a sore throat.
- Stop smoking.

WHEN TO CALL A HEALTH PROFESSIONAL

- If you cannot trace the cause of the sore throat, such as postnasal drip of a cold, low humidity, excessive yelling, etc.
- If someone in the family has recently had strep throat.
- If you have a history of frequent strep throats.
- If sore throat is accompanied by a fever of 103°.
- If mild sore throat lasts

more than 2 weeks (be-
comes chronic).
- If, on examination with a
penlight, the throat is very
bright red, or has white
spots or pus on it.
- If there is a foul odor from
the mouth.

Strep Throat

Strep throat is an infection caused
by a streptococcal bacterium which
can lead to rheumatic fever and possible rheumatic heart disease in 3%
of children and young adults who
get it. Strep infections can even occasionally lead to kidney disease.
Strep is a serious infection which
must be diagnosed and treated by a
health professional. It is usually accompanied by a moderately high
(103°) fever, bright red throat, pus
or white spots on tonsils or throat,
swollen glands and severe pain, and
sometimes by a foul odor from the
mouth. In an adult, there may be
only a low fever (99°).

Strep is very difficult to recognize
without a culture. Not infrequently,
the person has no symptoms other
than a mild sore throat. To take a
throat culture, a swab is brushed
against the back of the throat and
the tonsils. A good culture usually
requires enough pressure to gag the
patient, and it does hurt a bit. The
materials taken on the swab are
then placed on a culture plate and
incubated. It takes 24–48 hours for
the materials to "grow out" and be

identified as a positive or a negative
strep infection.

Even an experienced physician
trained in diagnosis cannot be sure
whether or not a sore throat is
caused by strep bacteria without a
throat culture. Therefore, if you
have a sore throat you cannot trace
to a specific cause such as low humidity or too much yelling or smoking, or if a sore throat with a cold is
more than minor, you should get a
culture. Also, the person with a history of strep should always be
checked, and if someone else in the
family has strep throat and you get
a sore throat, have yourself cultured. Sometimes the whole family
is cultured to look for a person who
might be an asymptomatic carrier.
(Someone with no symptoms who
carries the bacteria.)

With just a little practice, almost
anyone can learn to take a proper
throat culture, which could save
you time and money. If strep
throats are a frequent occurrence in
your family or if you face the need
of having the whole family cultured, investigate the possibility of
throat culture kits. You swab the
throat at home, place the swab in a
test tube, and cork the tube. It is
then cultured at your physician's
office or a laboratory. See Throat
Culture Kits, page 213.

HOME TREATMENT

- You must see a health professional whenever any bacterial illness such as strep

throat is suspected. An antibiotic, given either by injection or orally, is the usual treatment if the diagnosis is positive.

- Continue taking prescribed medication, unless it is making you ill, for the length of the time prescribed (usually 10 days). *Do not stop* even if you feel completely recovered. The full 10 days are needed to kill the bacteria and to prevent a quick recurrence of the infection.

Swollen Glands (*Lymph Nodes*)

The lymph nodes are small glands that swell and harden when infection occurs in the body. The most noticeable nodes are those in the neck. (For location of lymph nodes, see page 8.) The lymph nodes swell and reduce as the body protects against minor infections from colds, insect bites, or small cuts. More serious bacterial infections may cause the glands to greatly enlarge and become very firm and tender.

Once lymph nodes harden, they may remain hard long after the initial infection is gone. This is especially true in children, whose nodes can remain hard and visible for several weeks after a bad cold.

HOME TREATMENT

There is no specific home treatment for swollen lymph glands. Continue treatment of the cold or other infection causing them to enlarge.

WHEN TO CALL A HEALTH PROFESSIONAL

- If the nodes are large, very firm, and very tender.
- If enlarged lymph glands are associated with other significant symptoms of infection.
- If enlarged nodes appear without apparent cause and persist for 2 weeks or more.

Small hardened nodes that follow a child's cold or minor infection and are not tender can be observed without professional help. They should be reported at your next regular visit to a health professional.

Tonsillitis

Tonsillitis is an inflammation of the tonsils. Tonsils are lymph nodes located at the back of the mouth on each side.

Since lymph nodes filter infections, the tonsils are affected by any throat infection.

Symptoms of tonsillitis are tiredness, fever, and sore throat. The tonsils will be very dark and swollen and perhaps pussy or spot-

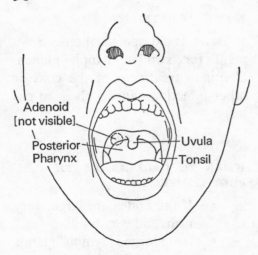

Adenoid
[not visible]

Posterior
Pharynx

Uvula

Tonsil

Location of tonsils

ted. The person sometimes vomits and may have a coated tongue.

A tonsillectomy (surgical removal of the tonsils) will only cure recurrent tonsillitis. It will not prevent colds or other infections. The infection will merely settle elsewhere. There are 2 main reasons to remove tonsils:

1. At least 4 recorded strep-tonsillitis infections in a year.
2. Abscess on the tonsils.

A tonsillectomy, like any surgery, is serious and carries some danger. The surgery should only be done for valid reasons after discussion with your physician.

HOME TREATMENT

- Tonsillitis requires the care of a health professional, who will probably take a culture to see if the infection is strep.
- Gargling with salt water may ease the pain of tonsillitis.
- Extra fluids will help dissolve the bacteria secretions and bring more healing blood to the area. Children and adults should drink a full 8-ounce glass every hour or so.
- Bed rest will help the body fight infection. Energy can then go to healing.

WHEN TO CALL A HEALTH PROFESSIONAL

- If there is a history of tonsillitis, especially several bouts per year.
- If a sore throat involves the tonsils and they are red, swollen, or pussy.
- If a fever over 103° accompanies a child's sore throat (101–102° for an adult).

6

A Rash of Skin Ailments

Skin problems affect most people at some time in their lives. Although they are rarely life-threatening, they can be a nuisance. Diagnosing skin problems may require the help of a health professional or a dermatologist (a physician specializing in skin problems), especially the first time you have a particular ailment. The second time it appears you should be able to recognize it and use home treatment. After diagnosis or recognition, refer to your individual problem listed alphabetically in this chapter.

Before you first meet with your health professional, try some general treatments for skin rashes to determine if the problem will clear up by itself. Wash the rash with soap and water and, if practical, leave it exposed to the air. Observe it and if it seems to get worse or to spread within 24 hours, call your health professional. Do not apply salves or ointments if the cause of

the rash is not known. The ointment itself might cause a reaction and perhaps make it more difficult for a health professional to discover the cause.

Any time a rash looks infected, call your health professional. An infection will be very bright red or pussy. Streaks of red leading away from the rash or from any skin infection are a more serious sign of infection.

If you have decided to call a health professional, first do a home physical exam. Then go through the questions below and answer those which pertain to your problem. Your answers will help you and your health professional in the diagnosis. You may even discover what is wrong on the phone.

A rash may sometimes be caused by emotional stress, tension, or nervousness. If stress appears to be a possible cause, review the relaxation techniques suggested in Chapter 12, page 204, and try to reduce the tension-causing events in your daily routine.

GENERAL PREVENTION OF SKIN PROBLEMS

One of the most important keys to good healthy skin is cleanliness. However, the skin can be washed too often. The body secretes natural oils to lubricate it. Soap and water wash these oils off, which is useful when there is excess oil, but harmful if the skin is dry. Too much soap and water can remove the protective lubrication causing dry, flaking, itching skin.

If you have dry skin, give some thought to whether you really need a shower twice a day or even daily, particularly in the winter months. Try bathing about 3 times a week with daily washings of the underarms, feet, and genitals. By eliminating a daily shower, you may be able to break the habit of washing off the skin's protective covering then putting on creams and lotions to replace it. If you really feel you need a daily shower but have dry skin, try a soap substitute which contains no detergent, or a mild soap without built-in deodorants. Your pharmacy will have many brands. Read the labels. It will be stated that it is a soap substitute.

Too many Americans have been convinced that human odors should be completely masked. The creams, lotions, sprays, and powders applied daily to the body as a human odor

---

Skin Rashes: History and Exam

Have you come into contact with something which irritates your skin? For a list of possible skin irritants, read about contact dermatitis on page 106–107.

Where did the rash first appear?

When did the rash appear?

Does this rash appear anywhere else on the body?

Is there a fever accompanying the rash? Record your temperature taken in the morning and at night.

Does the rash appear to have spread?

Does the rash itch? (Surprisingly, many do not.)

Does it hurt?

Does anyone else in the family have a similar rash?

What immunizations have you had?

Are you taking any new medication, either prescribed or over-the-counter?

Is there a sore throat with the rash?

Have you been under unusually heavy stress recently?

Have you been unusually nervous or tense?

---

replacement can harm your skin. They can be a source of an allergic reaction, causing itching, rashes, or infections. At any rate, soap and water are more effective than perfumed cover-ups.

Acne

Acne is the term for inflamed spots appearing over the face, back, and shoulders. It occurs most often in adolescence. Acne is caused by a number of things. Apparently, hormonal balance affects acne, and adolescence is the time when hormones are adjusting. Small skin follicles become plugged with oil and may cause irritation of the surrounding skin.

PREVENTION

- Cleanliness is essential. Hot soapy water and a washcloth are 2 of the best preventive tools. Use a backbrush for your back.
- Stress or anxiety seem to aggravate acne in some people, so worrying over acne probably only makes it worse. It is a difficult cycle that only you can stop.
- For years it was believed that diet played an important role in causing acne flare-ups. Teenagers were discouraged from eating nuts, chocolate, and other forbidden foods. Some doctors now feel that diet is not a significant cause of acne. Everyone is different, and if acne seems to occur after eating a particular food, avoid that food. It could be, however, that you are reacting to stress. You have heard for so long that a food is bad for your complexion that you become anxious whenever you eat it. Thus, anxiety rather than the food could be one source of the acne.

HOME TREATMENT

- Again, cleanliness is essential. Wash your face, shoulders, and back with soapy water and a washcloth 3 times a day. Use a backbrush. If your regular soap doesn't seem to help, try an over-the-counter soap manufactured for acne. Always rinse very thoroughly.
- Long hair seems to make acne worse. Consider keeping your hair shorter and off the forehead.
- Steam, or warm wet towels placed on the skin for 10–15 minutes 2 or 3 times a day will often help open the glands and allow for deeper cleaning.
- Sunlight and sun lamps sometimes help by drying the skin and allowing the outer layer to drop off, which opens some of the

plugged glands. Care should be used with a sun lamp. Protect the eyes and eyelids with goggles and keep the lamp 24 inches away from the face. Limit the first exposure to 1 minute. The desired effect will be mild redness and light peeling. Never go to sleep with a sun lamp on and always use some type of timer.

- Try to eliminate some of the tension in your life. See page 202 for ways to cope with tension.

WHEN TO CALL A HEALTH PROFESSIONAL

- Cases that cannot be controlled with the above suggestions should be seen by a physician.
- Some doctors prescribe oral antibiotics which have been known to cure acne. Even so, caution should be taken not to over-use antibiotics. You must decide whether or not curing your acne is worth the risk of antibiotic treatment. See the discussion of the appropriate use and dangers of antibiotics on page 227.
- Your health professional may also prescribe medication that is applied directly to the skin.
- If your acne continues to be

a real problem don't hesitate to see your doctor to discuss further therapeutic measures that may help.

Athlete's Foot

Athlete's foot is a fungal infection which is not restricted to athletes. Fungus is present everywhere, but grows best in warm, moist, dark places. Bare feet come in contact with wet surfaces where the fungus is present, such as in community showers. The fungus then thrives in tennis shoes or anywhere we perspire a lot and where air cannot circulate.

Symptoms include cracked and peeling areas between the toes and intense itching. If symptoms don't subside with the use of antifungals, then you may have an allergic reaction common to feet that perspire a lot.

PREVENTION

- Keep your feet clean and dry. If members of your family are susceptible to athlete's foot, use an antibacterial agent such as Lysol or Pinesol when cleaning showers. Wear thongs in a community shower such as a public swimming pool shower.

HOME TREATMENT

- Wear cotton socks to absorb perspiration.

- Consider changing your socks during the day to keep your feet dry.
- Alternate your pairs of shoes from day to day. This will allow your shoes to dry out completely between use so that they are less likely to harbor the fungus.
- Tinactin, Desenex, or Verdefam are fairly good antifungals available over-the-counter. They come in powder, cream, or spray form.

WHEN TO CALL A HEALTH PROFESSIONAL

- If you are a diabetic or if circulation to your legs is impeded, you should not try self-treatment but see a health professional. It is particularly important to avoid inflammation or infection if you have either condition.
- If the skin appears to get worse after you apply the antifungal, discontinue using it and see your health professional. You may be sensitive to the ingredients in the medication.
- If the infection continues and does not seem to be getting better. You may need a more powerful antifungal prescription.

Bald Spots

Bald spots should be distinguished from baldness. Nothing can be done about the natural tendency that some people have for baldness. It is hereditary and no potion or vitamin pill made at the present time will make your hair grow again. However, bald spots that occur on a normal scalp may not be natural occurrences and may perhaps indicate a more serious problem.

WHEN TO CALL A HEALTH PROFESSIONAL

- Bald spots with a gray-green scale are often ringworm. Ringworm of the scalp can be very difficult to cure. Seek your health professional's help.
- If you have bald spots, it is a good idea to call your health professional as this may be a signal of a variety of problems.

Bee Stings

Some people are more sensitive to bee stings than others. Most bee stings cause a localized reaction: the area stung will swell, redden, and itch. Sometimes this localized reaction will be quite severe and persist over a length of time, but it is not an allergy as long as it is still localized. An allergy to a bee sting is a reaction that is generalized throughout the body. There can be hives all over the body, shortness of breath, tightening of the throat muscles, or difficulty in swallowing. A very severe reaction can cause death. In fact, more people die annually as a result of bee stings than from snake bites.

PREVENTION

- Anyone who has had a generalized reaction or a severe local reaction to a bee sting should carry a bee sting kit. Such a kit can be obtained with a prescription and contains immediate treatment for bee sting reactions.
- People who have had a generalized reaction may also check into having a series of shots to desensitize them and prevent severe reactions to bee stings. This is a relatively new procedure and should be discussed with a health professional.

HOME TREATMENT

- For a localized reaction, use cool cloths or ice to relieve the pain. Antihistamines may be used if the itching is severe. See page 224 for Antihistamines.
- Bees leave stingers imbedded in the skin. Remove the stinger with tweezers. The localized symptoms should then decrease.

WHEN TO CALL A HEALTH PROFESSIONAL

- If a person has a generalized reaction *IMMEDIATE* professional help is needed. These signs are:
  - o Hives all over the body.
  - o Shortness of breath or wheezing.
  - o Difficulty in swallowing.
- To discuss obtaining a bee sting kit or getting the series of desensitization shots for a person who has had a generalized or a severe local reaction in the past.

Birthmarks

Birthmarks, which come in all sizes, shapes, and colors, usually disappear by themselves. The flat purple ones on the upper eyelids, lower forehead, and back of the neck and large, flat, bluish ones on the lower back will go away eventually. Brown, flat, oval birthmarks are there to stay and will do no harm. You can watch this type during regular home physicals and report to your health professional if they grow or otherwise differ from their normal appearance.

Strawberry birthmarks are lumps that can appear anywhere on the body. They usually appear after birth and enlarge during the first year of life. They become raised, red, and soft but most of them will disappear if they are left alone. They will start to recede after a year but will leave an area of skin that does not tan well. It is best not to have these removed surgically or any other way as the treatment is unnecessary. If surgery is necessary for cosmetic reasons, it is better to wait until the child is older and more cooperative.

WHEN TO CALL A HEALTH PROFESSIONAL

- For surgery if a birthmark is cosmetically unacceptable.

Boils

A boil is a red, swollen, painful area on the skin similar to an overgrown pimple. Boils occur most often in areas where there is hair and irritation, such as on the neck, armpits, genitals, breasts, face, and buttocks. A boil occurs when a hair follicle gets plugged and doesn't drain. This becomes a perfect place for bacteria to grow because the body fluids are trapped in that one place. The pus inside a boil is white blood cells that came to clear the infection away. Pain is caused by pressure on the nerve endings due to the swelling.

PREVENTION

- Do not scratch a boil that you already have. You might carry the bacteria to healthy areas of the skin and cause more skin infections.

HOME TREATMENT

- Bring moist heat to the area as often as possible. Soak a washcloth in very warm water and place it directly on the boil for 15 minutes. Keep the cloth warm by replacing it in the warm water whenever it gets cool. This moisture will keep the surface soft and free from scabs that might close the skin and trap the infection. The heat increases the blood flow to the area which promotes the healing process and brings the boil to a "head." This treatment is most effective when you first notice a boil.
- Cut fingernails so you cannot scratch the boil.

WHEN TO CALL A HEALTH PROFESSIONAL

Your health professional can surgically drain the boil or treat it with antibiotic drugs. See the discussion of the appropriate use of antibiotics on page 227. You should call a health professional if:

- The pain stops you from normal activities.
- You have a fever over 100°.
- No progress has been made

in 2–3 days of good soaking treatment.

Chicken Pox (Varicella)

Chicken pox is highly contagious and almost all children will get it. It is a relatively minor disease, however, and children do not usually become very sick. Chicken pox can occasionally lead to encephalitis, an inflammation of the brain. However, encephalitis usually subsides without complications.

Symptoms of chicken pox include a rash of red pimple-like spots that turn into clear blisters. The rash can cover the entire body including the throat, mouth, ears, genitals, and scalp. A child might also have just 1 or 2 spots. If anyone in the neighborhood or classroom has chicken pox, start looking for symptoms in your child in about 2 weeks. Chicken pox is contagious 1 day before the rash appears until all the pox are scabbed and dry. In the first couple of days, your child will be in generally ill health, and have a fever and abdominal pain. Then the blisters on the skin appear.

PREVENTION

- There is no useful prevention. In fact, the disease is less bothersome for a young child than an adult so some parents willingly expose their children. However, the severity of the disease has no relation to how close to an infected person a child is when exposed.

HOME TREATMENT

- Try to make the child comfortable.
- You will want to control the itching because if scabs are scratched off too early they may become infected. For itching relief treatments, see page 112.
- Cut the child's fingernails.

WHEN TO CALL A HEALTH PROFESSIONAL

- If there is fever over 102° that lasts for more than 2 days.
- If severe itching cannot be controlled by aspirin and warm baths.
- If bruising appears without injury.
- If sores are in the eyes.
- If you notice signs of encephalitis that can occur after any viral infection. These signs are:
  o Severe headache
  o Unusual sleepiness
  o Continued vomiting

Contact Dermatitis

Contact dermatitis is a skin rash that occurs because the skin has touched a substance which causes an allergic reaction. Any rash that

Contact Dermatitis History Chart

When did the rash first appear?

Where did the rash appear?

Does the rash appear anywhere else on the body?

Have you changed shampoos or hair dyes lately?

Does the rash involve that part of your body where clothes are worn?

Have you changed detergents lately?

Any new jewelry?

Have you been near plants such as poison oak, sumac or poison ivy?

Any new hand cream or nail polish?

Any new medications taken recently?

appears only on a specific localized part of the body is likely to be contact dermatitis. Poison ivy, laundry soaps, and jewelry are all common sources of contact dermatitis although hundreds of other items may cause irritations in certain individuals.

If you have a localized rash, try to discover the possible source of irritation. Above are the types of questions you can ask yourself. The list is not an exhaustive checklist of irritants, but merely a starting point for your history taking process. You are best able to fit the questions to your lifestyle. Your list of questions should start with the location of the rash. A foot rash, for example, would probably relate more to new shoes or socks than it would to your new shampoo.

HOME TREATMENT

- If you do discover the cause of the rash, remove the irritant.

- Wash the rash with your usual soap and water because a new soap may cause another rash.
- If practical, leave the rash exposed to the air.
- For itching relief treatments, see page 112.

WHEN TO CALL A HEALTH PROFESSIONAL

- If the rash becomes infected. This means that it is very bright red or pussy.
- When fever is 101° or more.
- If there are red streaks leading away from the rash.
- If after 2 weeks you have not discovered the cause of the rash and it still continues to bother you. In this case, answer the questions in the Dermatitis Chart and any others you can think of before calling your health

professional. Your health professional will ask the same questions to discover the irritant. You will save time and aid in discovering the cause of the rash if you have given thought to the questions in advance.

Cradle Cap

Cradle cap is a thick scaling or greasy crusting, like dandruff, common to many babies. It is often caused by not washing an infant's head well enough for fear of damaging the skull during a bath. A baby's skull is not that delicate and can be regularly and thoroughly washed to prevent cradle cap. If you see some crusting or discoloration of the scalp, you are probably not washing vigorously enough.

HOME TREATMENT

- Give the baby's head a good scrubbing with a washcloth or soft brush and your regular baby shampoo. Scrub hard. You can also try loosening the scales with baby's comb before shampooing.
- If scrubbings with regular shampoo don't work, try using Ionil T, Sebulex, or Selsun Blue shampoos. Use caution when applying these as they are not baby shampoos and will irritate your baby's eyes.

Dandruff

Dandruff occurs when the skin cells of the scalp flake off. This flaking off is natural and occurs all over your body. On the scalp, however, flaking can cause problems by mixing with oil and dust to form dandruff.

Although dandruff cannot be cured, it is often necessary to control it.

HOME TREATMENT

- Try frequent and energetic shampooing with any shampoo. Hair can be shampooed daily and should be if this controls your dandruff.
- If the dandruff is excessive and itchy, you might try a dandruff shampoo. Experiment, then use the one that works best for you. Some brands to try include Selsun Blue, Sebulex, Ionil T, and Tegrin.

WHEN TO CALL A HEALTH PROFESSIONAL

- If shampooing frequently doesn't seem to control dandruff. Your health professional might prescribe a dandruff shampoo.

Diaper Rash

Diaper rash is a reaction to the ammonia in babies' urine, to their stools, or to the soap used to wash diapers. While it is uncomfortable, diaper rash is usually not dangerous.

Symptoms of the rash are a red bottom and thighs. It will be easier for you to recognize this after you have seen it the first time.

PREVENTION

- Try to change the diapers as soon as possible after they have been soiled or wet.
- Leave the skin open to the air as often as possible.
- Don't wash the diapers in too much soap.
- Make sure the diapers are rinsed well after they are washed thoroughly.
- Avoid using the lined disposable diapers or plastic pants for a while, if your baby has frequent problems. These trap the moisture and keep it against the baby's skin.

HOME TREATMENT

- Every baby is unique, so try a few different methods to find out what is best for your baby.
- Wash your baby's skin around the diaper area thoroughly with plain soap and water and then dry the skin well.
- Change diapers frequently.

Don't use excessively bulky or multilayered diapers.

- Add 1 ounce of vinegar to 1 gallon of rinse water.
- You can try protecting the skin with Desitin, Diaperene, or zinc oxide.
- Sometimes cornstarch or baby powder on the diaper area will be more comfortable. If you do use powder, be sure to put it in your hand first as shown, rather than sprinkling it right on your baby. You and your baby will inhale less powder this way.
- Stop using plastic pants when the rash appears.
- Try changing detergents if the rash does not clear.

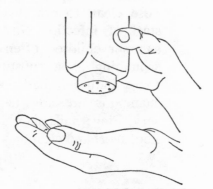

Applying powder

WHEN TO CALL A HEALTH PROFESSIONAL

- If the diaper rash becomes very bright red.
- If the rash becomes raw or sore looking.
- If the rash has blisters or crusty patches.

Impetigo

Impetigo is a bacterial infection which often starts when a small cut or scratch becomes infected. Symptoms are oozing, scabbed, honey-colored, crusty sores. These sores usually appear on the face between the upper lip and the nose. However, impetigo spreads easily so it may appear anywhere on the body. Bacteria gets under the fingernails and is spread by scratching.

PREVENTION

- Washing all scratches with soap and water is one of the best ways to prevent impetigo. If your child has a runny nose, keep the area between the upper lip and nose clean to prevent the start of infection. In the summer children often go swimming as a substitute for a bath but baths and shampoos are still necessary. Fingernails should be kept short and clean.

HOME TREATMENT

- If one honey-colored crusty sore appears, try scrubbing it with soap and water. Bacteria grows under the scabs so scabs must be removed. Twenty minutes of soaking every 2 hours followed by gentle soapy scrubbings should remove the scabs. You can give

warm soaks on the face by using a warm washcloth. When the washcloth becomes cool, rinse it in warm water.

- Dry the skin without rubbing the sores. Try using a hand-held hair dryer after light towel drying.
- Follow the soapy scrubs with application of an over-the-counter antibiotic ointment such as Neosporin, Neo-polycin, or Neomycin. Sometimes the fluids oozing from the lesion will lift the ointment. In this case it would be better to use a cream which would mix with water.
- If one person in the house has impetigo, the other members are susceptible to the infection because it spreads easily. Try to insure against this spreading by:
  o Having each member of the household use separate washcloths and towels.
  o Not having anyone share the same bath water.
- Men should not shave over the sores but around them. Use a new razor blade daily and do not use a shaving brush.
- *DO NOT* put adhesive bandages on the sores. The adhesive applied to the skin

provides a warm shelter for the bacteria to multiply. Also, when the adhesive is pulled off, it pulls dead skin with it. This creates new entry points for the bacteria to invade. If you must cover the infection, use gauze and get the adhesive as far away from the infection as possible.

WHEN TO CALL A HEALTH PROFESSIONAL

- If you cannot seem to make any progress in controlling impetigo and any new crop appears. Your health professional will be able to prescribe an antibiotic to clear it up.
- If the area around the nostrils, face, and/or lips swells and becomes tender.
- If there is red streaking leading away from the infected area or there is pain in a nearby lymph gland.
- If the infected person gets sick and has a fever over 101°.

Ingrown Toenails

Ingrown toenails most often occur on the big toe. The nail gouges into soft toe tissue causing pain, inflammation, and infection. This usually results from trimming the nails too

short, especially at the corners. Shoes which are too tight or an injury to the toe might be other causes of ingrown nails.

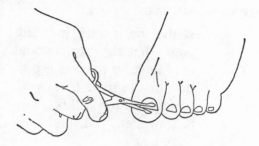

Cutting toenails

PREVENTION

- Cut your toenails straight across rather than rounding them. Be sure to leave the corners of the nails long enough to prevent gouging.
- Buy roomier shoes if yours are too tight.

HOME TREATMENT

- Soak your foot in warm water. You should then be able to draw the nail away from the toe far enough to place a wisp of cotton between the nail and the toe. This will cushion the area where the nail is gouging. This procedure should be done daily until the corner of the nail has grown beyond the point where it cuts into the flesh. It is not necessary to replace the cotton daily; leave the first one in place throughout all soakings, checking to make sure it's there daily.

- If the toe is very infected, your health professional may have to remove a portion of the nail. If it is infected, the toe will be painful, swollen, red, and may ooze pus.

Itching

Itching accompanies many skin rashes. Since for most diseases it is advisable not to scratch the skin, you need to know how to relieve itching. The first two methods below seem contradictory but try these to see which works best for you.

HOME TREATMENT

- Keep the area cool and wet. Try cool compresses or a compress soaked in Burrows solution available at the drugstore.
- Try to relieve itching with warm water. Wet a cloth in water as hot as you can stand (120–130°) and apply it for a few seconds.
- Baths with ½ cup of baking soda in a tub full of warm water sometimes relieve itching.
- Apply cornstarch or bak-

ing powder pastes to the skin.
- Try to forget about the itching by putting your mind on other things. Games may keep a child's mind off the itching.
- Alpha-Keri and Syntex are bath oils which are excellent for dry, itching skin, but use them very sparingly.
- Try an over-the-counter antihistamine such as Chlor-Trimeton.

WHEN TO CALL A HEALTH PROFESSIONAL

- If itching is very severe a stronger antihistamine may be prescribed for relief.

Jock Rot or Jockey Itch (Tinea Cruris)

Jockey itch is a fungal infection that occurs in the groin area of males and females. This fungus grows best in warm, moist places.

Symptoms include severe itching and moistness in the genital area and thighs. There are red, raised areas on the skin which may also weep or ooze pus or liquid.

PREVENTION

- People who perspire a lot are susceptible to jockey itch, especially if they do not bathe often enough to wash away the perspiration. You should wear cotton underpants to absorb perspiration, bathe often, and keep your clothes clean.

HOME TREATMENT

- Rub cornstarch over the genital area after bathing. This will dry the infection and prevent friction.
- Wear cotton underpants.
- Avoid pants that are too tight and cause friction.
- Bathe often.
- If you have a more severe case, try an over-the-counter antifungal such as Verdefam, Tinactin, or Desenex.

WHEN TO CALL A HEALTH PROFESSIONAL

- If the above treatments do not seem to be working, you might need an antifungal prescription.

Lice

Lice are small, white, wingless insects about the size of tiny ants that live on the human body. They can live on anyone's body and in the past few years there has been a huge increase in the cases of lice infestation. The adult is called a louse and its eggs are called nits. Nit-picking, then, is the removal of the louse eggs, a tedious task since the nits are so small.

There are 3 types of lice: head, body, and crab. Head lice appear on the hairs of the head, behind the ears, and on the back of the neck. To check for head lice look through the hairs; lice or nits should be seen along the hair shafts. Body lice are rarely seen as they inhabit the seams and lining of clothing and move to the body only when feeding. Crab lice infest the groin and pubic area.

Lice suck blood. However, it is their saliva and excreta which cause you to itch. Lice are spread by close contact with such things as car seats, coat racks, theatre seats, combs, sexual contact, and bedding. Head lice are very common in school children since they are in such close contact. They are rapidly transmitted on coat racks.

The main symptom of lice is itching. You should also be able to see the nits, which adhere to a hair shaft.

HOME TREATMENT

- Kwell and Eurax are prescription shampoos and are highly effective in getting rid of lice. Cuprex and A-200 Pyrinate are over-the-counter remedies that will usually do the job. Shampoo the entire family and thoroughly clean the clothing, bedding, rugs, and furniture in your home. You may need to boil things to sterilize them or iron those things you cannot boil. Repeat this treatment in 48 hours to kill the lice that hatch from eggs already laid.

WHEN TO CALL A HEALTH PROFESSIONAL

- If you tried over-the-counter remedies and were not successful, you can discuss whether a prescription for Kwell or Eurax is needed.
- Call your public health department and they will assist you both in treating the problem and in preventing reinfestation.

Measles

There are 2 types of measles: Rubeola (called red, regular, 2-week, or hard measles) and Rubella (called German, 3-day, or soft measles). The symptoms of these 2 diseases are quite different so they will be discussed separately. However, prevention for both is the same.

PREVENTION

- Every child should be immunized against both types of measles. The MMR (measles, mumps, Rubella) immunization is available and effective. In the 1940s, an immunization for measles was made from a dead virus. It has long since been discovered that this type will not provide life-long immunity. Anyone given this type of vaccine was also given an additional shot of gamma globulin at the same time. If you or a family member were given this type of vaccine you should be revaccinated with the live virus.

Rubeola (Red Measles or Regular Measles)

Regular measles can be serious and is very contagious. Symptoms appear 8–12 days after exposure. Initial symptoms are fever, runny nose, hard dry cough, and red eyes. After a few days a spotty rash will appear and the fever will rise and continue until the rash has covered the body. The rash appears first on the face and neck, and covers the whole body within 3 days. These spots will later fade from the head down. The disease is contagious from just before the rash appears and will continue to be contagious while the rash remains.

Encephalitis, or inflammation of the brain, is a possible complication of regular measles. Protect your child from measles and any complications by immunization.

HOME TREATMENT

- Give plenty of liquids.
- Humidify the room to help the dry cough.

- Limit television viewing and reading books as the eyes are unusually sensitive.

WHEN TO CALL A HEALTH PROFESSIONAL

- If any sore throat occurs, especially with a rise in fever. This could be strep throat.
- If the temperature is nearly normal for 2 days, then rises above 101°. It is possible that a secondary infection has developed.
- If difficulty in breathing occurs. This could be a sign of pneumonia.
- If the child has a convulsion.
- If an earache develops.
- A blue, gray, or purple color to the lips or beneath the nails might indicate pneumonia.
- Thick, discolored mucus out of the nose could be a sinus or ear infection developing.

Rubella (*German, Three-day, or Soft Measles*)

Rubella is a relatively minor disease in a child. It is contagious for 1 week before the rash appears. Symptoms occur 14–25 days after exposure and include a mild, low-grade fever, muscular aches and pains, and occasionally a headache. The lymph glands in the neck may swell and the eyes may be slightly inflamed. A rash of tiny pimples will then appear, usually first on the face and neck. The rash will cover the whole body in 12–24 hours. Rubella usually lasts 3 days.

Rubella is a dangerous disease when a woman contracts it during the first 3 months of pregnancy, since it can cause severe fetal damage. An adult woman can be tested to determine if she has immunity to Rubella. If a woman who has not had Rubella wishes to start a family, she should discuss vaccination with her health professional. Some health professionals are reluctant to immunize since a woman shouldn't become pregnant for at least 3 months after vaccination.

HOME TREATMENT

- To relieve itching, see page 112.
- Avoid any exposure to a woman who could possibly be pregnant.

WHEN TO CALL A HEALTH PROFESSIONAL

- If the patient appears to becoming sicker and sicker each day.
- When fever is greater than 102°.
- If patient has convulsions.
- If patient is extremely listless or lethargic.

Mosquito Bites

A mosquito bite appears as a red, raised bump. While not dangerous, itchy mosquito bites can be a real nuisance.

PREVENTION

- Good insect repellents are very effective in preventing mosquito bites. Apply them to all exposed areas of the skin and thin clothing whenever a lot of mosquitoes are around. Reapplication every few hours may be needed. Be sure to protect your infant by applying a repellent or by keeping the child covered when you are in an area that has many mosquitoes. Your pharmacist can recommend a good repellent like Off, 6–12 Lotion, or Cutters. Prevention is especially important if there are reported cases of mosquito bite-caused encephalitis in your area.

HOME TREATMENT

- To relieve itching, see page 112.
- If the bite is bothersome because it swells a little, apply a cool compress.
- Trim the fingernails of children to prevent them from scratching and infecting the bites.

Moles

Pigment gives skin its color. When the pigment is close together it is called a mole. Moles are sometimes raised and hairy and appear more on some people than others. Heredity may play a part in the number of moles you have, as parents with moles tend to have children with moles. They appear throughout a person's life and during pregnancy and adolescence may tend to darken and enlarge.

Moles are rarely pre-cancerous. Actually, a mole has about the same chance of becoming cancerous as any other part of your skin.

HOME TREATMENT

- Become familiar with your own moles. Know their normal color, shape, and size so that you will be aware if they change.
- It is okay to pluck offensive hairs from a mole.
- You can remove a mole at home. Reasons for removal include:

    It offends you because you feel it harms your appearance.

    An article of clothing is rubbing against the mole and continually irritates it or causes it to bleed.

    To remove a mole, tie a thin string such as dental floss around it after pulling it away from the skin with blunt nose tweezers. Tie the string tightly to cut off the blood to the mole. In a couple of days the mole will be dried up and will fall off. After that, watch it to make sure there is no infection.

WHEN TO CALL A HEALTH PROFESSIONAL

- If a mole changes in size or color by darkening or lightening.
- For removal if you don't feel you want to try home removal or if the mole is flat and you can't get a string around it. Also have a mole removed by a health professional if it has been changing in size or color, because it should be analyzed after professional removal.

Prickly Heat or Sweat Rash

Prickly heat, also called miliaria or sweat rash, is a rash consisting of single or multiple red dots that appear over an infant's head, neck, and shoulders. These dots look like tiny, white-headed pimples.

Prickly heat is often caused by well-meaning parents who dress their baby too warmly, but it can happen to any baby in really hot weather. An infant should be dressed just as lightly as an adult and will be comfortable at the same temperature. Babies' hands and feet feel cold to your touch because

most of their blood is near the stomach helping digestion.

PREVENTION

- Do not over-dress your baby. You can tell if a baby is too warm by placing your hand between the shoulder blades. If the skin is hot or moist, the baby is too warm.

HOME TREATMENT

- Dress the baby lightly.
- Cornstarch or powder will make the baby more comfortable.

WHEN TO CALL A HEALTH PROFESSIONAL

- If the rash seems infected.
- If the infant has a sick appearance.
- If the rash persists over 3–4 days.
- If sweat rash is accompanied by a fever of 101° that doesn't come down after you remove warm clothing.

Psoriasis

Psoriasis is a chronic skin disease that affects about 6% of the population in the United States. It appears as silvery skin patches which are often on the knees and elbows although they can be anywhere on the body. In a normal person the outer layer of skin cells is replaced every 30 days. In a psoriatic the outer layer is replaced every 3 or 4 days. The silvery patches, called plaques, are composed of dead skin cells which accumulate in layers.

PREVENTION

- Psoriasis seems to be partly hereditary. It is *not* contagious so there is no fear of "catching" it.

HOME TREATMENT

- There is no known cure for psoriasis although there may be remissions and rarely the disease may disappear completely.
- Sunlight seems to be one of the most effective treatments. Sunbathe often, but avoid sunburn.
- The therapeutic value of the sunlight can be increased if you apply a photosensitizing tar preparation containing 5% coal tar distillate such as Tar Doak. Tar Doak is an over-the-counter drug. Apply it 20 minutes before exposure to the sun. Remove excess before sunbathing. The disadvantages of using a tar preparation are that it sometimes causes inflammation of the hair follicles and may stain the skin and look unattractive.
- For moderate scalp scaling

try tar shampoos such as Sebutone, Zetar, or Polytar shampoos.
- Try to reduce some anxiety and tension in your life. These can cause outbreaks or increase severity of outbreaks. See page 202 for ideas on how to relieve stress.

WHEN TO CALL A HEALTH PROFESSIONAL

- See your health professional for a diagnosis if you suspect psoriasis. Your health professional may prescribe topical steroids or other forms of therapy.
- If it is generalized, that is, covers much of your body.
- If you experience joint pain.
- If the psoriasis gets worse despite home treatment.

Ringworm

Ringworm is a fungal infection of the skin. It develops into a red, scaly, itching ring which can appear anywhere on the body. Ringworm of the scalp may appear gray and is hard to diagnose.

PREVENTION

- Ringworm is frequently transmitted to people by cats which carry the fungus. If your family adopts a cat, have it checked for ringworm by your veterinarian. Teaching your children not to snuggle with stray cats with bald patches is wise, but they may still contract the disease from cats which have ringworm buried beneath their fur.

HOME TREATMENT

- Try Desenex or Tinactin, both over-the-counter drugs, on small spots.

WHEN TO CALL A HEALTH PROFESSIONAL

- If ringworm is severe and spreading, a prescription is probably needed.
- If there are spots on the scalp, especially if the hair is missing.

Second, if penicillin is incorrectly prescribed at the onset of the fever, the child could be incorrectly diagnosed as having a penicillin allergy when the rash occurs.

HOME TREATMENT

- Lots of liquids.
- Lower the temperature as you would for any high fever to reduce the risk of convulsions, i.e., sponge bath, aspirin, or acetaminophen.
- If a convulsion occurs, see treatment on page 81.

WHEN TO SEE A HEALTH PROFESSIONAL

- See the same warning signs under convulsions, page 81.

Roseola

Roseola infantum is a rose-colored rash. Called just roseola, it is a viral infection usually seen in babies 6 months to 3 years of age. The disease often starts with a sudden high fever (103–105°) and irritability. The fever continues for 2–3 days, then as it drops a red rash which looks like measles appears on the face and trunk. The rash fades in 24 hours.

Two things are worth noting about this disease. First, there is a slight possibility of convulsions occurring since the fever is so high.

Scabies

Scabies is caused by tiny mites which burrow into the skin. They cause severe itching which starts about a month after being infested. The mites are seldom seen for they live in the burrows they make under the skin. You can acquire scabies either by direct contact with an infected person or by actual physical contact with clothes, bedding, etc., of an infected person.

The key symptom of scabies is severe itching. Your skin will have tiny bumps, burrows, and tunnels that look like exclamation marks.

These can be found on the genitals, breasts, in the armpits, along the belt line, or between the fingers.

PREVENTION

- Promptly treat any symptoms of scabies to prevent spreading.
- General cleanliness will prevent scabies.
- Since scabies infestations are highly contagious, wash more thoroughly and more frequently, especially if you have had recent contact with an infected person.

HOME TREATMENT

- Wash all bedding and all clothing articles and iron the mattress to kill the eggs of mites. It is important to kill not only the mites but eggs to prevent further infestation. The entire household must be treated at the same time or else eggs will be left in clothing or bedding to start the cycle again.
- Kwell lotion, a prescription, must be applied to all household members.

WHEN TO CALL A HEALTH PROFESSIONAL

- To discuss whether a prescription for Kwell is needed.

Scarlet Fever

Scarlet fever is a strep throat with a rash. It is not as prevalent today as it once was and, once contracted, can be treated with antibiotics.

Symptoms of scarlet fever include a high fever and a rash formed with pinhead-sized dots which are prominent over the cheeks, chest, abdomen, and groin. The skin appears "sand papery." The little bumps on the tongue get bigger and redder, making the tongue appear to have a strawberry or raspberry texture. In many cases, about 10 days to 3 weeks after the illness the skin peels.

PREVENTION

- Scarlet fever is spread through contact with an infected person. Avoid people with a known case of the fever.

WHEN TO CALL A HEALTH PROFESSIONAL

- If a rash accompanies a sore throat.
- If a rash peels and the child has had a sore throat in the recent past, see a health professional. Even if the child seems well and is peeling, it is worth having a throat culture taken. If the culture indicates strep, antibiotics will be prescribed to cure the strep throat infection.

Skin Cancer

Skin cancer is the most common of all cancers. Fortunately, it is also the form of cancer we know most about. Most skin cancer is caused by prolonged and frequent exposure to the sun. In fact, 90% of all skin cancer occurs on the face, neck, and arms where exposure to the sun is most frequent. Fishermen, farmers, construction workers, and others who spend much time out-of-doors are very likely to develop skin cancers along with a very leathery complexion. Lighter skinned, blue-eyed people are also more likely to develop skin cancer than those who normally tan easily. Black people run little risk of skin cancer.

Skin cancer doesn't usually develop until middle age or later. Even so, solar damage to the skin in early life will greatly contribute to skin cancer later.

Fortunately, most skin cancers are slow growing and are easy to recognize and treat long before they reach a serious stage. Virtually all of these slow growing cancers can be completely cured by simple, inexpensive removal in a physician's office.

A small percentage of skin cancers are much more serious. Such cancers, called malignant melanomas, can quickly invade the body and spread to other body tissue. Melanomas, unless treated quickly, may often lead to death.

PREVENTION

- Skin cancer can be prevented by reducing skin exposure to the damaging rays of the sun. Loose-fitting, light-colored clothing is effective in blocking most of the damaging ultraviolet rays. For exposed areas the only effective protection is the regular use of sunscreens. Sunscreen creams, foams, lotions, and oils are able to screen out up to 90% of the harmful rays.

Sunscreens should not be confused with the many suntan lotions which do little to stop the ultraviolet light. Sunscreens with the ingredient PABA are particularly effective. Examples are Presun, Sundown, and Sure Tan Sunscreen. Read the label before you buy. Although sunscreens allow a person to get a light golden tan, they prevent the burning and dark tanning that lead to premature aging and skin cancer.

HOME TREATMENT

- Once skin cancer has developed, nothing can be done at home to treat it. Home emphasis should be placed on preventing further cancers by using sunscreens and other protective measures.

- If a pigmented mark or elevation appears or changes size or color.
- If a scaly blemish persists, bleeds, or changes in character.
- If a sore persists without healing for 4–6 weeks.
- If a wart or mole changes in size or color.

Sties

A sty is a little pimple or small boil that appears on the edge of the eyelid. It will usually come to a head and break, then go away. The problem with a sty is that it contains pus germs which can be easily transmitted to other parts of the eye causing more sties.

HOME TREATMENT

- Wash hands after touching a sty to prevent spreading.
- Application of moist heat for 20 minutes every 2 hours will help the sty either come to a head or disappear. Use a washcloth that has been soaked in very warm tap water.

WHEN TO CALL A HEALTH PROFESSIONAL

- If the sty becomes larger, more tender, or painful.

- If more than one sty appears.

Sunburn

A sunburn is usually a first-degree burn which involves just the outer surface of the skin. Sunburns are uncomfortable but usually not dangerous unless they are extensive. They are, however, quite dangerous if extensive in infants or small children.

PREVENTION

- There is really no good excuse for getting a sunburn since there are excellent creams available which screen out the sun's burning rays but still allow a tan. Over-the-counter products containing PABA are good. Examples are Sundown, Presun, or Sure Tan Sunscreen. Sunscreens should be reapplied periodically, especially after swimming.

HOME TREATMENT

- Watch sunburned children or infants for signs of dehydration. See page 30 for dehydration symptoms.
- Cool baths can be very soothing.
- A low-grade fever and a headache can accompany a sunburn. Lie down in a

cool, quiet room to alleviate the headache.

- Drink lots of water and eat some salty crackers to replace fluid and salt loss.
- Sucking on ice chips will help control nausea.
- There is nothing you can do to prevent peeling; it is part of the healing process.
- Watch for signs of heat exhaustion. See symptoms on page 153.

WHEN TO CALL A HEALTH PROFESSIONAL

- If there is severe blistering.
- If there is a fever of 102° or more.

Ticks

A tick is a small insect that fastens itself to the body. A tick should be removed as soon as you discover it. It can detach itself readily from you voluntarily but if you try to force it off, you may break off its mouth parts and they will remain embedded in your skin. You will cut the risk of infection if you do not leave any parts behind.

HOME TREATMENT

- When camping you should check daily for ticks. This check includes both you and your pets.
- When you return home

from camping or hiking make a thorough check for ticks.
  - o Check the scalp by feel while shampooing.
  - o Check the rest of the body visually.
- Methods of removing a tick:
  - o Light a match, blow it out, then immediately touch the glowing end to the tick. This might convince the tick to back out.
  - o An ice cube might work.
  - o A drop of household oil such as 3-in-1 dropped on the tick might make it come out as would any substance that would smother it, even peanut butter!

WHEN TO CALL A HEALTH PROFESSIONAL

- If a fever or infection develops after a tick has been removed.
- If you are unable to remove the entire tick.

Warts

Warts are growths on the skin that are caused by a virus. They can appear anywhere on the body but usually on hands and the backs of fingers. Warts are not dangerous but can be very bothersome.

Little is known about warts. We don't know where they come from, what makes them go away, why a treatment will work one time but not the next, or why some people seem to be more susceptible than others. So if you seem to have found a cure for your warts, keep on using it. The following guidelines in Home Treatment may also be helpful.

HOME TREATMENT

- Warts appear and disappear spontaneously. They can last a week, a month, or even years. To get rid of your warts, you have to believe in the treatment. Faith and incantations seem to work just as well as faith and over-the-counter preparations.
- If the wart bleeds a little, stop the bleeding with a little pressure.
- If the wart is in the way, for example when you are writing, use a pumice stone or a mild ointment containing 5% salicylic acid. Both of these are over-the-counter products.
- Plantar warts appear on the feet and can be painful. You can buy doughnut-shaped pads made of foam rubber which alleviate the pressure on the wart when

you walk. If a pad does relieve the pain and the wart doesn't increase in size, use it. Otherwise, see your health professional.
- Try the least expensive method of treating warts that you can think of and you may save a trip to your health professional.
- Don't attempt to cut or burn off a wart yourself.
- Warts often go away if you simply ignore them!

WHEN TO CALL A HEALTH PROFESSIONAL

- Your health professional can remove warts by freezing them, by electrolysis, with chemicals, or by cutting them off. The removal of warts, however, may leave a scar so you should try home treatment first, unless:
  o The wart has been irritated or knocked off. It could then become infected.
  o A plantar wart is painful when you walk and is not relieved by the foam pads.
  o The wart causes discomfort.
  o The wart is cosmetically unappealing.
- Warts will often re-appear even after professional removal.

7

Injuries

Few of us make it through a year without some kind of minor injury. And it sometimes seems a child can't make it through a whole day without at least one "owwie." If you know how to treat these minor injuries, you can save money and unnecessary visits to your health professional.

When children are injured you'll often need to deal with both the injury and the anxiety and fear which it may cause. In adults, too, reassurance and understanding are medically important parts of injury care. Try to approach injuries with a matter-of-fact attitude which recognizes the pain or problem and expresses understanding and support.

You can usually treat injuries with a minimum of tools. For example, the best treatments for bruises, strains, sprains, and burns is something almost everyone has, and it's free. Ice. A small paper cup filled with water and put in your freezer is a quick source of ice, which reduces swelling and unnecessary pain. The paper cup of ice can be used for small injuries by peeling away some of the paper and exposing some ice. Be sure any time that you apply ice that you keep it moving all over the wound, "painting" the wound. If you don't, skin tissue may be damaged by the ice.

Accidental Tooth Loss

If a permanent tooth is lost because of an injury, a dentist may be able to re-implant it in the mouth. A baby tooth probably cannot be re-implanted and has to come out anyway, so it isn't worth the effort to save it. However, sometimes when a baby tooth is lost prematurely, the permanent teeth will grow in crooked in order to fill the gap. Call your dentist to determine if a spacer is needed to temporarily fill the space left.

HOME TREATMENT

- Wrap the tooth in a piece of wet gauze or place it in a small glass of salt water.
- Immediately call your dentist for an emergency visit.

WHEN TO CALL A HEALTH PROFESSIONAL

- To re-implant the tooth. The sooner you get to a dentist, the better the chance the tooth will stay in. Your odds are best if you see a dentist within the hour the injury occurs. After 24 hours there is little chance the tooth can be successfully re-implanted.
- If the tooth lost was a baby tooth to determine if a spacer is needed.

Animal Bites

The main concern for most people when they have been bitten by an animal is whether or not a rabies shot is needed. The main carriers of rabies are wild animals, especially skunks, bats, rats, and squirrels. Rarely do pet cats and dogs have rabies since most have been immunized at least once. If a pet has bitten you, it needs to be observed for 10 days to see if it develops symptoms of rabies. If the owners cannot be relied on to watch the animal, call the dog warden to catch and quarantine it.

Bacterial infections are common in animal bites that break the skin. Tetanus can occur if shots are not up-to-date.

PREVENTION

- Don't try to catch wild animals or provoke them to attack.
- Don't rush up to a dog without making sure it is friendly. It should be wagging its tail and not snarling or growling.
- Observe beware-of-dog signs.

HOME TREATMENT

- If the bite doesn't require a rabies shot, clean the wound thoroughly with soap and water. Treat it as you would a puncture wound (see page 138) if the skin has been penetrated, and watch for signs of infection.

WHEN TO CALL A HEALTH PROFESSIONAL

- If rabies shots may be needed. Below are some reasons a shot should be considered:
  o Any wild animal bite.
  o If the animal was a domestic cat or dog but is acting strangely, foaming at the mouth, or is very thirsty.

o If the animal owner has no record of the pet being vaccinated for rabies.

o If the bite has penetrated the skin and your tetanus shots aren't up-to-date. See page 233 for a schedule of tetanus shots.

Blood Under a Nail

Fingernails and toenails often get crunched, bashed, or smashed. These injuries usually aren't too serious but when swelling under the nail occurs it can be very painful. The injury causes bleeding but there is no soft tissue between a nail and bone to absorb the blood so it is trapped under the nail. Pressure builds and causes pain.

The throbbing and pain can be relieved only by draining off the blood. To do that, you need to make a hole in the nail. This can be done at home rather than in a health professional's office. You may feel squeamish about trying this method, but it is the same thing a health professional would do.

HOME TREATMENT

- As soon as possible after the injury, apply ice. This will minimize the swelling.
- If pressure and pain require a hole to be made in the nail, follow these steps:

o Straighten a paper clip and heat the tip in a flame until it is red hot. You'll need a flame like a match or a gas burner rather than the rods of an electric burner.

o Place the tip of the paper clip on the nail and let it burn through. This will not be painful as the nail has no nerves. A tough nail may take several tries.

o As soon as the hole is complete, blood will escape and the pain will be relieved. Absorb the blood with the tip of a handkerchief or a piece of gauze.

o If the pressure builds up again in a few days, repeat the procedure, using the same hole.

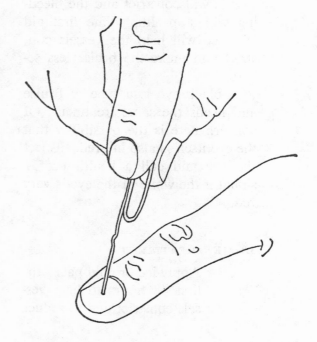

- If the victim is really un-cooperative and won't let you try the procedure.
- If the nail appears infected. The nail is infected if it is red, hot, or has pus under it.

Bruises (Contusions)

When your body is battered or bumped, a bruise develops. A bruise is caused by a blow which ruptures small blood vessels. The vessels bleed into the soft surrounding area. When the blood doesn't have enough oxygen, the cells turn from red to blue which causes the color of a bruise. The area will either keep bleeding until the tissue can't hold any more blood, or the vessels will constrict and the bleeding will stop. Immediate first aid with ice will help the vessels constrict and make the bruise less severe.

A black eye is a type of bruise and needs the same treatment. Of concern here is the possibility that the eye itself is also injured. Inspect the eye and call a health professional if the white of the eye is very red.

HOME TREATMENT

- Apply ice or cold packs the first 48 hours to help vessels constrict and to reduce the swelling. The quicker you apply ice after the injury the less bleeding will result.
- If possible, elevate the bruised limb. Blood will leave the area of the wound and there will be less swelling.
- Rest the limb so you won't injure it further.
- If the area is still painful after 48 hours, apply heat with warm towels, a hot water bottle, or a heating pad.

WHEN TO CALL A HEALTH PROFESSIONAL

- If signs of infection develop. The symptoms are:
  o increasing severe pain
  o fever of 101° or more
  o marked swelling and surrounding redness
- If the bruise is a black eye and the white of the eye is very red.

Burns

Burns are classified as first, second, or third degree depending on their depth, and not on the amount of pain or the extent of the burn. A first degree burn involves just the outer surface of the skin. The skin is dry, painful, and sensitive to touch. A mild sunburn is an example. A second degree burn involves the tissue beneath the skin in addition to the outer skin. The symptoms are swollen, puffy, weepy, or blistered skin. A third degree burn involves the outer skin, tissue beneath the skin, and any underlying tissue or organs. The skin is dry, pale white or charred black, swollen, and sometimes broken open. Nerves are destroyed or damaged so there may be a little pain except on the outer edges where there is a second degree burn.

PREVENTION

Some major burns would be less severe if the fire were extinguished quickly. If you catch on fire, roll over and over on the ground to smother the flames. If another person catches on fire, roll the victim in a blanket, rug, or coat to stifle the flames. If the victim is allowed to run, air will fan the fire and make it worse. If a hose is handy, use it to put out the flames. This will cool the burned areas and reduce the severity of the burns.

TREATMENT

For minor burns:
- For treatment of sunburn, see page 122.
- Ice or cold is the best immediate treatment for minor burns. The cold lowers the skin tempera-

ture and lessens the severity of the burn. Immediately run cold tap water over the burn. While you do this, send someone to get some ice. Ice in a paper cup can be applied directly to a burn if you keep the ice moving around. The application of ice hurts for a while but it is the best treatment.

- Do not put any salves, butter, grease, oils, or lubricants on a burn. They don't do any good and can irritate the skin more.
- There is no need to cover the burn unless it is rubbing against clothing. If it does rub, however, it is better to cover it than to break open the blisters. To cover such a burn, remove any burned clothing. Wash the burned area and cover it with a single layer of gauze. Tape the edges of the gauze well away from the burned area. This dressing needs to be changed the following day and then every 2 days.
- Shock is often present with major burns especially if they involve the head, face, hands, feet, or genitals. See page 160 for prevention and treatment of shock.
- A third degree burn needs immediate medical treatment. Do not apply any

salves or medication since these will have to be removed later for treatment and their removal may be harmful.

- If a burn involves the face, hands, feet, or genitals.
- If the pain lasts over 48 hours.
- For all third degree burns.
- If an infection starts developing. Signs of infection are:
  o Fever of 101° or more
  o Pain and swelling increase
- If in doubt as to extent of burn or in doubt if it is a second or third degree burn.

Chemically Burned Eye

Chemical burns to the eye occur when something caustic, such as window-cleaning fluid, gasoline, or turpentine, is splashed into it. The eye appears reddened and watery.

If the damage is more severe the eye appears whitish.

HOME TREATMENT

- It is important to immediately flush the eye with ordinary tap water to dilute the chemical. The most effective way to do this is to fill a sink or dishpan with water, immerse the face of the victim in the water, and then open and close the eyelids to force the water to all parts of the eye. It may sometimes be necessary to move the eyelids with the fingers.
- Keep dunking under water until the eye stops hurting.

WHEN TO CALL A HEALTH PROFESSIONAL

- If after 20 minutes of Home Treatment, the eye still hurts.
- If the eye appears to be damaged. Symptoms include:
  o persistent redness
  o discharge
  o watering
  o any visual impairment such as double vision, blurring, or sensitivity to light

Are Sutures Necessary?

SUTURES NEEDED:

- The wound is deep and tends to gape widely.
- The cut is deep and is located on a part of the body that bends and puts stress on the cut. Examples of such stress areas are elbows, knees, and fingers.
- A cut on the scalp tends to separate and usually needs stitches.
- Deep cuts on your thumb or palm of your hand may cut nerves affecting your sense of touch.
- A slit lip needs suturing because it scars easily.
- Cuts to eyelids need stitches to prevent drooping.
- Whenever you are particularly worried about scarring, especially with facial cuts. A sutured cut usually heals with less scarring than an unsutured one.
- Cuts that go down to the muscle or bone.
- If bleeding, even from a minor wound, cannot be controlled with 20 minutes of direct pressure.

SUTURES NOT NEEDED:

- Cut edges of the skin tend to fall together.
- Cuts less than 1 inch long that aren't deep.

Cuts (Lacerations)

What concerns most of us when we see a cut is whether or not stitches or sutures are necessary. In general, stitches are used to hold the 2 edges of a wound together so that healing can occur with a minimum of scarring. The chart above gives more specific guidelines as to whether or not you need to have a cut sutured.

If a cut doesn't need stitches, be sure to bandage it properly at home. Always put an adhesive strip on a cut crosswise rather than lengthwise. This will bring the edges into firm contact and promote healing.

To remove an adhesive bandage, pull it slowly in the direction of hair growth to prevent pain caused by pulling against the hairs.

A butterfly bandage, very useful in holding together cut skin edges, can be made at home or purchased. The adhesive is on the outside edge so the middle part over the cut isn't sticky. To make a butterfly bandage follow the steps below:

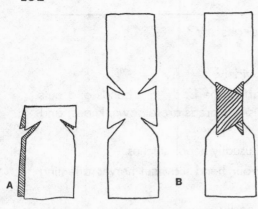

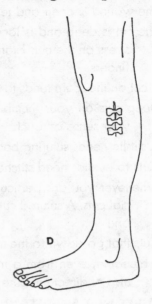

- If the cut is long, you may need to use more than 1 bandage as in part D.

The butterfly bandage

- Cut a strip from a roll of 1 inch adhesive tape and fold it sticky-side out. Cut wedges into the tape as shown in part A.
- Unfold the tape then fold the wedged pieces together sticky-side in as in part B. The center of the tape will not now be sticky.
- Place one end of the tape on the skin, then pull the other end to tightly close the wound as in C.

HOME TREATMENT

- Wash the cut with soap and water.
- Stop the bleeding by applying pressure. See page 145.
- Use a regular adhesive strip or butterfly bandage to continue the pressure.
- There is no need to use antiseptics such as iodine, mercurochrome, or merthiolate. These can harm delicate tissues and slow healing.

WHEN TO CALL A HEALTH PROFESSIONAL

- If you feel the cut may need to be sutured.

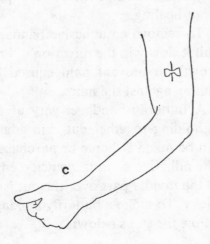

- If the cut becomes infected. Symptoms of infection are:
  - o increasing pain
  - o tenderness
  - o swelling
  - p fever of 101° or more
  - o red streaks leading away from the wound
  - o redness around the cut

Fishhook Removal

Sometimes in the excitement of fishing, fingers are hooked instead of fish. It is convenient to know how to remove a fishhook by yourself, or for a fishing companion, especially if you are far from medical help.

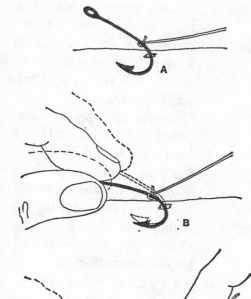

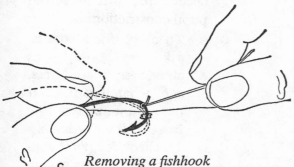

Removing a fishhook

HOME TREATMENT

- Remove the hook by the following steps:
  - o Use cold, or hard pressure to provide temporary anesthesia.
  - o Tie a piece of fishline to the hook near the skin surface. See part A below.
  - o Grasp the eye of the hook with one hand and press down about ⅛ of an inch to disengage the barb. See part B below.
  - o While still pressing the hook down (barb disengaged), jerk the line parallel to the skin surface with the other hand so that the hook shaft leads the barb out of the skin. See part C below.
  - o Wash the wound thoroughly. Use soap if any is available.

WHEN TO CALL A HEALTH PROFESSIONAL

- Puncture wounds are susceptible to tetanus infection. See page 233 for a discussion of whether a tetanus shot is necessary.
- If the wound becomes infected. Symptoms are redness, pus, or heat from the area of the wound.

Freeing Trapped Limbs

Often fingers, arms or legs get caught in objects such as bottles, jars, or pipes. This happens to children and adults alike. It is most important to stay calm at these times, because panic will only make the situation worse.

HOME TREATMENT

- Don't start forcing the limb. This will only make it swell and become more difficult to remove.
- Try to get the victim to relax the limb. Relaxation alone will sometimes enable you to free the limb.
- If possible, elevate the limb.
- Apply ice around the exposed limb. Hopefully, this will reduce any swelling that has already occurred and allow the limb to be released.
- If ice doesn't work, dribble dishwashing soap or oil down the limb. Turn the limb or the object so you are sort of screwing it out rather than pulling it directly out.

Head Injuries

Head injuries are frightening and can be very serious because of the potential for brain damage, but not every head injury involves a concussion or brain injury.

There are certain steps to follow when someone suffers a blow to the head which will help you decide whether a health professional should be seen.

HOME TREATMENT

- Treat the injury as you would any injury. Stop the bleeding, clean, and bandage the wound. Check for other injuries.
- A blow to the head may cause a lot of swelling and a lot of bleeding. This is not *necessarily* serious.
- After a few moments, when the person has calmed down, ask some questions to see if he or she is confused. Ask name, address, what day it is, etc.
- Observe the person frequently for the next 24 hours. *Immediately following the injury and every 2 hours for the next 24* (set your alarm during the night) do the following checks for alertness and pupil constriction:
    o To check for alertness, ask questions, as above: name, address, age, what day it is. If the person appears confused, call a physician.
    o To check for pupil constriction: Using a pen-

light in a darkened room, direct the light from the side into each pupil, several times. If the pupils do not constrict, or one constricts considerably more than the other one, call a physician immediately. See page 6 for more information on pupil constriction test.

WHEN TO CALL A HEALTH PROFESSIONAL

- If the person has lost consciousness at any time following the injury.
- If the person is very confused after the first few minutes following the injury.
- If there is nausea and vomiting *after* the first 2–3 hours following the injury. Limited nausea or vomiting at first is normal.
- If there is violent, persistent vomiting after the first 10–20 minutes.
- If the pupils do not constrict or do not constrict evenly. This indicates an *immediate* call.
- If the person has a loss of memory of more than a minute.
- If there is double vision.
- If there are seizures, similar to a convulsion.
- If there is weakness or numbness on one side.

Insect in the Ear

Getting an insect in your ear can be a pretty frightening experience, especially for a child. It is sometimes difficult to know if an insect is in the ear rather than something else. Your child may say, "My ear is bumping around," or you may see the bug. Once you know for sure that it is an insect there are a couple of tricks you can try to get it out.

HOME TREATMENT

- Don't try to kill the insect by poking something in the ear, because it will be much more difficult to get out.
- Insects are attracted to light so may be coaxed out with light. If you are outdoors, pull the earlobe gently to straighten the canal and aim the ear towards the sun. If indoors, shine a flashlight into the ear while pulling gently on the earlobe. Hopefully, the insect will crawl out toward the light.
- If the light method fails to work, dribbling a little mineral oil into the ear may cause the insect to float out. You must be *sure* that it is a bug in the ear before trying this method. If it is a bean, popcorn, or something similar, the object may swell and be difficult to remove.

WHEN TO CALL A HEALTH PROFESSIONAL

- If neither of the above methods work.
- If you decide that it is something other than an insect in the ear.

Nosebleeds

Nosebleeds can be inconvenient and messy, but they can be stopped with home treatment. Causes of nosebleeds range from lack of humidity to a fractured skull. Some common causes are the ordinary cold, allergies, blows to the nose, medication, high altitudes, blowing the nose, a foreign object in the nose, and low humidity.

PREVENTION

When a nosebleed occurs, try to figure out what caused it. You may save yourself from future occurrences by eliminating the cause. An example of this is a nosebleed caused by low humidity. Humidifying your house or at least the sleeping areas and turning the heat down to 60–64° may prevent future nosebleeds.

HOME TREATMENT

- Pinch the nostrils shut between your thumb and forefinger for 5 full minutes. Watch the clock as you're doing this. Don't let go after a couple of minutes to see if it's still bleeding or you will have to start timing yourself again. The victim should be seated during the treatment, not lying down. Also, hold the head erect rather than tilted backwards. Blood will run down the throat and may cause choking if the head is leaning backwards.
- After 5 minutes, release the nose. If it is still bleeding, hold it for another 5 minutes.
- After the bleeding has stopped, insist the victim stay quiet for a few hours. This means no blowing of the nose, no loud talking, and no laughing.

WHEN TO CALL A HEALTH PROFESSIONAL

- If the bleeding hasn't stopped after 3 tries of 5 minutes each.
- If the bleeding was caused by a fracture of the nose. Suspect a fracture if there is a deformity in the outline of the nose.
- If nosebleeds keep occurring and you can't find the cause.

Object in the Eye

Sometimes something gets in an eye that tears can't remove. If the speck is under your upper lid, you can learn to evert or "flip" the lid to ease removal. This method is described in Home Treatment below.

HOME TREATMENT

- If the speck is in the side of the eye or by the lower lid, moisten the tip of a twisted piece of tissue and touch the speck with the end. The debris should cling to the tissue.
- If the object is under the upper lid, you may need to flip the lid.
  - o Ask the victim to look down at the floor.
  - o Grasp the eyelashes and pull the lid away from the eyeball.
  - o Place a cotton swab or wooden match stick across the outer surface of the lid near the lashes.
  - o Pull the lid forward and upward which will cause the lid to roll and fold back over the applicator. The lid will now remain rolled up and won't need to be held.
  - o If the speck is on the eyelid, remove it with a moistened cloth or tissue.
  - o When you are through, the victim can look at the ceiling to allow the lid to drop back in place.
- If the object has scratched the eyeball, put a patch on that eye to prevent the eyelid from flickering and further irritating the scratch. An indication that the eyeball has been scratched is if there is still pain after the object has been removed.

Flipping a lid

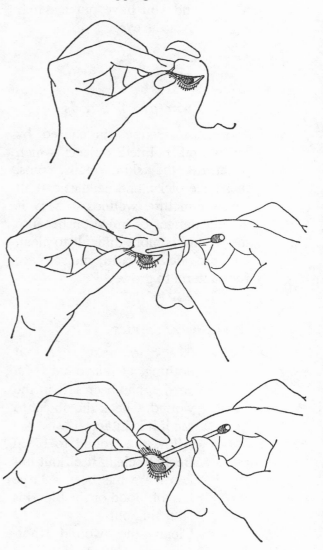

- If the object is on the eyeball rather than on the eyelid. You could damage the eye if the object severely scratches the eyeball. This is especially true if an object has penetrated the eyeball at all.
- If you cannot remove the object yourself.
- If pain persists 2–4 hours and you have put a patch over the eye.

Puncture Wounds

A puncture wound is caused by sharp and pointed objects which penetrate the skin. Nails, pins, tacks, ice picks, and needles can all cause puncture wounds. There is greater danger of infection because the wound is more difficult to clean and provides a warm, moist place for bacteria to grow.

HOME TREATMENT

- Check to make sure that nothing, such as the tip of a needle, has been left in the wound. Check the object to see if it is intact.
- Allow the wound to bleed freely to clean itself out unless there has been a large loss of blood or the blood is squirting out.
- Clean the wound thoroughly with soap and water.
- For the next 4–5 days, soak the wound several times a day in warm water. This will keep the wound open to allow it to heal from the inside out. If the wound is closed, an infection beneath the skin may not be detected for several days.

- If the wound is in the head, chest, or abdomen, unless it is obviously minor.
- If the wound shows signs of infection, such as:
  o fever of 101° or more
  o pus or increased redness
  o swelling
- If the source of the puncture wound was dirty such as barbed wire, a rusty nail, or a farm implement, you need a tetanus shot if yours isn't up-to-date. See page 233 for a discussion of whether or not a shot is necessary.

Recognition of Fractures

Fractures and sprains often mimic each other. Both are painful and shouldn't have any weight put on them. Sprains can be treated at home, as described on page 140. Fractures need to be seen by a health professional. When you do have a fracture, *call* your health professional rather than rushing to the emergency department of your hospital since they will have to call your doctor anyway. There is usually no immediate need to treat a fracture as long as it is immobilized and swelling can be kept at a minimum. See Splinting, page 140. A Sunday night broken finger can wait for treatment on Monday if initial treatment is started—reduce the swelling and don't use the finger.

The following symptoms may be helpful in recognizing a fracture. X-rays will usually be needed to confirm the diagnosis.

WHEN TO CALL A HEALTH PROFESSIONAL

- If the limb is obviously bent out of shape or a bone is poking through the skin.
- If the limb is twisted unnaturally.
- If the victim can't move the injured limb.
- Run your finger along the bone line. If you feel an irregularity it could be a fracture.
- *Gently* press the area of the injury. Pain is often centered at the site of a break. Pain from a sprain may be more spread out.
- If there is a *lot* of swelling and discoloration.

- If you are uncertain of the nature of the injury and the pain continues or increases.

Scrapes (Abrasions)

Scrapes or abrasions happen so often that they seem unimportant. They need to be treated, however, to reduce the chance of scarring or infection.

HOME TREATMENT

- The worst thing about scrapes is that they are usually very dirty. You need to remove all dirt and debris to prevent scarring and possible infection. Use a pair of tweezers to remove obvious pieces of debris, then scrub vigorously with soap and water and a washcloth to clean the wound. If you have a vegetable sprayer in your kitchen sink, try using that on the scrape with additional scrubbing. The victim will probably complain loudly of the pain, but remember that you are preventing scarring.
- You may apply an antibiotic ointment, but it isn't a necessity. Neosporin and Mycitracin are a couple of over-the-counter examples.
- If the scrape is rather large, cover it with a non-stick bandage. This type of bandage won't stick to the

scrape and is held in place by adhesive around the edges. Telfa is an example. If you apply a bandage and wish to use an ointment, put the ointment on the bandage, then the bandage on the scrape. This will be less painful.

WHEN TO CALL A HEALTH PROFESSIONAL

- If the scrape becomes infected. Signs of infection are:
  - o swelling
  - o increased pain
  - o red streaks leading away from the wound
  - o pussy discharge
  - o fever of 101° or more

Splinting

Splinting is used to immobilize a suspected fracture to prevent further injury. Anything that's close at hand that will prevent the injured part's moving can be used as a splint.

There are 2 general ways to immobilize an injury: wrapping something around the injured limb, or tying the limb to some other part of the victim's body. For the first method you can use newspapers, magazines, an umbrella, a stick, a cane, or anything else that is stiff. Tie whatever you have to the injured limb with a rope, a belt, torn strips of cloth, or anything else con-

venient. Position the splint so that the injured limb cannot bend. A general rule is to splint a joint above and a joint below the fracture. The second method includes taping one broken toe to a healthy one and immobilizing an arm by tying it across the victim's chest.

Sprains and Strains

A *sprain* is an injury to the muscle, ligaments, tendons, and soft tissues in the region of a joint. Ligaments, tendons, and small blood vessels are stretched and sometimes torn when a joint is sprained. A *strain* is a muscle injury from overexertion or stretching. Because treatment for both injuries is the same, they are presented here as one type of injury. For treatment of back strains specifically, see page 57.

HOME TREATMENT

- If the sprain is to a finger or other part of the hand, immediately remove all rings. They may have to be cut off later if swelling occurs.
- Do not put weight on the injured joint. This can cause further damage. A sprain is just as painful as a fracture and needs just as much care. For a badly sprained ankle, use crutches. The inconvenience of crutches is justified by the faster healing of the ankle.
- Immediate application of

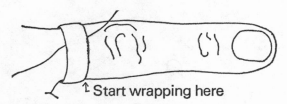

↥ Start wrapping here

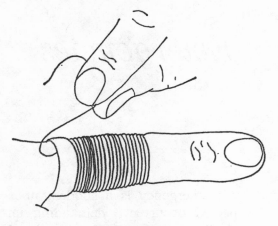

Removing a ring

ice or cold packs is needed to prevent or minimize swelling, especially for wrists and ankles. For difficult-to-reach injuries, use an ice bag or wrap ice cubes in a towel. Apply ice for up to 48 hours after the injury.

- If possible, elevate the injured limb while applying the ice treatment to decrease the swelling.
- Wrap the injury with an elastic bandage. This helps to immobilize the sprain to prevent further damage. Be sure to loosen the bandage if swelling occurs and the bandage becomes too tight or uncomfortable.
- After 48 hours of cold treatment switch to heat. A hot water bottle, warm towels, or a heating pad will speed up the healing process but do not apply anything that is uncomfortably warm.
- If you did not remove the ring before the swelling started, try the method below to remove it:
  o Stick the end of a slick piece of string under the ring toward the hand.
  o Starting at the knuckle side of the ring, wrap the string snugly around the finger toward the end of the finger, wrapping beyond the knuckle. Each wrap should be right next to the one before.
  o Grasp the end of the string that is stretched under the ring and start unwrapping it, pushing the ring along in place of the unwrapped string until the ring passes the knuckle.

WHEN TO CALL A HEALTH PROFESSIONAL

- If the injury appears to be a fracture rather than a sprain. See Recognition of Fractures on page 138 for symptoms of a possible broken bone.
- If the sprain is not improving after 4 days of home treatment.

8

Emergencies

An emergency is a sudden, unexpected occurrence demanding immediate action. Unfortunately, it can also be a time for panic and fear. We all dread coming upon an emergency and not knowing what to do. If you take the time to learn what to do now, you will be better able to cope during an emergency.

The most important thing to remember in any critical medical occurrence is to stay calm. By staying calm, you can better assess the situation and help the victim relax. This relaxing can help the victim by slowing bleeding, improving breathing, and easing pain.

The next step in any emergency is to identify and prioritize the injuries. Carefully examine the victim. If the person is unconscious, check the pulse and respiration rates. Then look for bleeding, broken bones, and signs of shock. The most serious and life-threatening injuries will have to be treated first. While a cut on the head can produce a lot of

blood and seem very serious, it is *relatively* unimportant if the patient is not breathing.

If you are needed in an emergency give what assistance you can. Most states have a Good Samaritan law that protects people who help in an emergency in good faith. You cannot be sued for administering first aid or medical care unless it can be shown that you are guilty of gross negligence. Your local law enforcement office can tell you what protection your state's laws provide.

A mental health emergency occurs when a person fails to cope adequately with any crisis which may lead to attempted suicide. The crisis can be caused by the death of a loved one, the threatened loss of a spouse, the loss of a job or income, the diagnosis of a terminal disease, or anything that upsets the person's normal functioning. When a person's normal coping skills are overburdened by such a crisis, anxiety and despair may arise. Anxiety symptoms following any crisis are a good indication that that person needs special help and support either from family and friends or from a mental health professional. A medical emergency occurs if help is either inadequate or too late to prevent a suicide attempt.

Most emergencies can be prevented. Look at your way of life and eliminate situations which endanger your family's lives.

lances are equipped with lifesaving equipment. If an ambulance is called unnecessarily, money is wasted. The ambulance may also be needed elsewhere for a more critical emergency. Children can be frightened by an ambulance ride and should be spared the experience if possible. However, if an ambulance isn't called when needed, a life may be lost. Use the chart below to help you decide if an ambulance is necessary.

Ambulance Usage

It's difficult to decide whether or not to call an ambulance in a medical emergency. Ambulance crews today are highly skilled and ambu-

Artificial Respiration

Breathing is a vital life function. Breathing may stop as a result of drowning, electric shock, suffoca-

---

Should an Ambulance Be Called?

CALL AN AMBULANCE IF:

- You are alone with the victim. It is impossible for you to drive a car and care for another person.
- You or the victim is having symptoms of a possible heart attack. These symptoms are severe chest pain, sweating, or shortness of breath.
- You suspect a spinal or neck injury. See page 58 for symptoms of these injuries.
- The victim is having severe breathing difficulty.
- There is severe bleeding. Have someone else call for help while you continue to apply pressure to the wound.
- You cannot cope with the emergency.

NO NEED TO CALL AN AMBULANCE IF:

- The victim is conscious, breathing without difficulty, acting normal and has strong vital signs, and there is someone else to ride in the car to give comfort to the victim as you drive. An example of this situation is when a child has a suspected broken bone but otherwise appears normal.

---

tion, drug poisoning, or other causes. All injured persons should be examined to see if they have stopped breathing or are having difficulty breathing.

To check for breathing look at the chest and abdomen to see if they are moving. Put your cheek next to the victim's mouth to feel air passing through the lips. If none of these signs is present, the victim is not breathing.

The most effective method for giving artificial respiration is mouth-to-mouth. It is explained in Home Treatment.

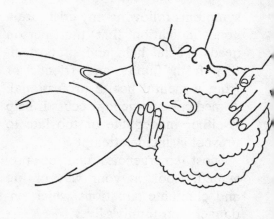

HOME TREATMENT

- Place the victim flat, face up.
- Turn the head to one side and clear the mouth of any foreign material with your fingers. Draw the tongue forward away from the back of the throat.
- Open the airway by pushing down on the forehead and lifting up on the neck. This position is shown opposite, top.
- Pinch the victim's nostrils shut with your hand still on the forehead and place your mouth over the victim's, making a tight seal. Blow in air until the person's chest rises. For an infant place your mouth over the nose and mouth. Blow with gentle puffs, just until the chest rises.

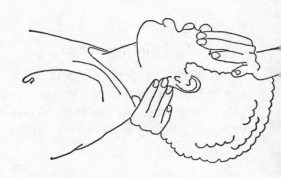

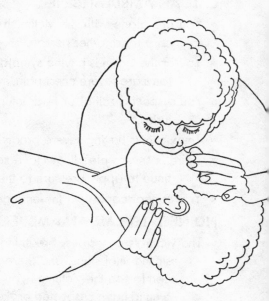

Artificial respiration

- Remove your mouth and allow the air to come out of the victim's lungs.
- Blow air into the lungs 12–15 times a minute on an adult and 20–30 times per minute for an infant.
- Discontinue when breathing is restored.
- Watch for symptoms of shock (see page 159).

WHEN TO CALL A HEALTH PROFESSIONAL

- Someone should call for medical help while you are performing artificial respiration.
- A revived victim still needs to see a health professional. This is important because a person can easily go into shock when breathing has stopped.

Bleeding

Severe bleeding from major blood vessels is referred to as hemorrhage. Since even small amounts of blood loss can cause shock, it is important to stop bleeding as quickly as possible.

HOME TREATMENT

- Most bleeding can be controlled by direct pressure for 10 minutes. It is best to use a folded, clean cloth or

towel, but if nothing else is available, use your bare hand. Find the place that is bleeding the most and concentrate your pressure directly on that area. It is important to maintain steady pressure for a full 10 minutes without peeking under the cloth or dabbing at the wound. If blood soaks through the cloth, apply another cloth without lifting the first. After applying direct pressure for 10 minutes, bandage the wound with the cloth still on to continue the pressure. If the wound is large, a firm bandage will be needed.

- If there is any ice available, apply some to the area surrounding the wound, but not directly on the wound. This should slow the blood outflow and speed the clotting process.
- If the bleeding is from an arm, hand, leg, or foot, elevate the injured limb as you apply pressure. Gravity will then help by not allowing as much blood to rush to the wound.
- As you control bleeding, look for and treat shock. See page 159 for the symptoms of shock.
- Tourniquets should be used only for severe, life-threatening wounds. This method is dangerous and

the victim's limb may be unnecessarily sacrificed. Virtually all bleeding can be stopped by direct pressure although sometimes it's necessary to press very hard or to apply a tightly wrapped bandage over the dressing. Make sure that direct pressure cannot stop the bleeding before resorting to a tourniquet.

WHEN TO CALL A HEALTH PROFESSIONAL

- If a cut requires stitches. See Cuts, page 131. Stitches are sometimes necessary to control bleeding that direct pressure cannot stop, even in small cuts.
- If a small cut continues to bleed through bandages after 20 minutes of direct pressure.
- If the victim has gone into shock, even if the bleeding has stopped. See Shock, page 159.

Blunt Abdominal Wounds

Blunt abdominal wounds caused by a blow to the stomach can cause severe bruising of the abdominal wall and internal bleeding from the abdominal organs. Such injuries are often caused by automobile, bicycle, tobogganing, and skiing accidents where the victim is thrown into something or to the ground.

The symptoms of abdominal injury are similar to those of external bleeding. Signs of shock will be present such as a rapid pulse, low blood pressure and cold, clammy skin. The abdomen may become rigid or tender. The victim may become confused and unable to recognize or describe the injury.

HOME TREATMENT

- Home treatment for an abdominal injury is limited to making the victim comfortable and observing the symptoms. Watching the victim's pulse and blood pressure are the best indicators of serious internal injury.

WHEN TO CALL A HEALTH PROFESSIONAL

- If abdominal pain, tenderness, rigidity, or signs of shock develop up to 48 hours after a blow or injury to the abdomen. Internal bleeding from an abdominal injury can become a serious emergency. Should you have any question about the symptoms you observe, call a health professional without delay.

Cardio-pulmonary Resuscitation (CPR)

Cardio-pulmonary resuscitation is required when the heart has stopped beating. If begun quickly and done correctly, it can restart the heart, prevent irreparable brain damage, and most importantly save a life. Thorough knowledge of how to do CPR will insure that it is done correctly and only when necessary.

The first thing to do when you encounter a person who has collapsed is to determine whether or not the person is conscious. Do this by firmly grasping the victim's shoulders and shouting, "Are you okay?" If the victim may have suffered a spinal injury be careful not to flex or twist the neck. Check this type of victim by digging your knuckle into the top of the breastbone, pinching them, or shouting at them to see if they react. If the person does not respond, you must check for breathing.

If you put your cheek next to the victim's mouth, you might feel air passing through the lips. At the same time look at the chest and abdomen to see if either is moving. If neither of these signs are present, the patient is not breathing and you should proceed to open the airway.

When someone stops breathing, the airway is blocked by the base of the tongue in the throat. To open it, make sure the victim is lying face up, then lift the neck with one hand and push down on the forehead with the other. See page 144.

After opening the airway, try to determine if the victim's heart is beating by locating the carotid artery. Find the voice box or Adam's apple, then slide the tips of your index and middle fingers into the groove beside it. Hold the fingers in place for 5–6 seconds so a slow or weak pulse is not missed. If the heart is beating at all, do not attempt CPR. The CPR compressions can damage a beating heart. If you determine there is no breathing but there is a pulse, do artificial respiration according to the instructions on page 144.

If you determine that there is no breathing *and* no pulse, it is time to start cardio-pulmonary resuscitation. CPR includes both compressions of the heart and intermittent mouth-to-mouth respiration. By applying rhythmic pressure on the lower half of the victim's sternum, you force the heart to pump blood.

It is difficult to perform CPR effectively without some instruction and practice on a mannequin. The best way to learn is to take a CPR class from your local Heart Association or Red Cross Chapter. Improper CPR techniques can cause injury, some very serious. Therefore, it is essential to be certain CPR is needed before beginning and then to do it properly. However, when a person's heart has stopped and there is no one trained at hand, then even if you aren't properly trained, give CPR to the best of your ability. The victim will surely die if you don't.

NOTE: CPR should *not* be practiced on people. Enroll in a CPR class where CPR mannequins are used for training and practice purposes.

The following steps illustrate the correct way to perform CPR:

1. Place the victim on a hard surface and open the airway.
2. Kneel at the victim's side, near the chest. Blow 4 quick breaths into the mouth.
3. Feel the chest to locate the lower tip of the sternum or breastbone.
4. Place the *heel* of one hand over the shaded area, about 1 to 1½ inches above the bottom tip of the sternum.
5. Place your other hand on top of the one that is in position. It sometimes helps to interlock your fingers. Do not allow your fingers to touch the chest as that may cause undue damage to the ribs.
6. Push down with a quick, firm thrust. You should push hard enough to press the lower portion of the breastbone down 1½ inches.
7. Now lift your weight from the victim, then repeat the compression and relaxation *once per second*. DO NOT lift your hands from the victim's chest during the relaxation.
8. If you are alone with the victim, give 2 mouth-to-mouth breaths after 15 compressions. If there are 2 rescuers, give 1 breath after 5 compressions.

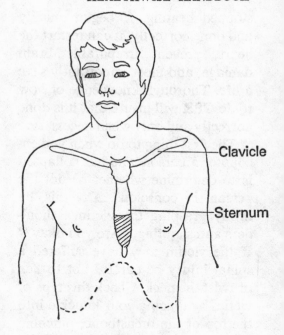

Location of sternum

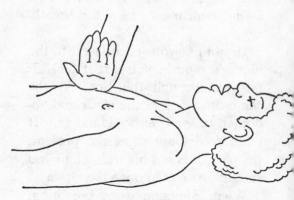

Placement of hand on sternum

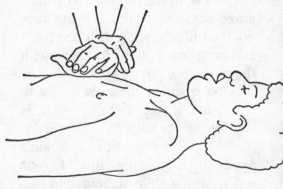

Hand position to avoid rib damage

9. *Do not pause during CPR for more than 5 seconds.*
10. Discontinue and check pulse if the victim shows any signs of revival.

Extra care is needed when giving CPR to infants and small children. An infant's neck is so flexible that when opening the airway you must be careful not to tilt too far backward, thus blocking the airway or damaging the spine. When using mouth-to-mouth breathing on a small child use 1 small breath every 3 seconds to inflate the lungs. For cardiac compression on infants use only the tips of the fingers of 1 hand when applying pressure and only depress the breastbone ½ to ¾ inches. On small children use the heel of 1 hand for compression and depress the breastbone ¾ to 1½ inches depending on the size of the child.

Chest Pain

To most people chest pain signifies a heart attack. Although chest pain is the best warning of a heart attack, there are different types of pain that may indicate other problems.

If you have chest pain that increases when you press your finger on the pain, you probably have chest-wall pain. This pain can be caused by muscles, ligaments, or bones in the chest wall.

A shooting pain that lasts only a few seconds is common and is no need for concern. Also a quick pain that occurs at the end of a deep breath is usually trivial.

Chest pains can be associated with other disorders. The pain from pleurisy gets worse with a deep breath or cough; heart pain doesn't get worse. An ulcer can cause chest pain and is worse on a empty stomach. Gallbladder pain often becomes worse *after* a meal.

WHEN TO CALL A HEALTH PROFESSIONAL

- Any chest pain associated with:
  o Sweating
  o Difficulty in breathing or shortness of breath
  o Fever of 101°
  o Nausea
  o Dizziness
  o Irregularity of the pulse
  o Pain that radiates to the arm, neck, and jaw

- Any chest pain that increases in persistency, frequency, or intensity.
- Any chest pain in someone who has a previous history of a disease associated with chest pain, such as a heart attack or a blood clot in the lung.
- Any chest pain that is constant and nagging and is not relieved by a change in position.
- Chest pain that lasts longer than 2 days.

Choking

An estimated 4,000 people choke to death on food every year. If you learn the simple technique for dislodging food caught in the throat, you may someday save a life.

The victim of a food choking is usually laughing and eating at the same time and then inhales a piece of food into the windpipe. A choked victim can't breathe, can't talk, and turns blue. If you don't take immediate action this person can have permanent brain damage in 3–4 minutes and can die in 4–8 minutes.

The technique used to remove a piece of food from a choked victim's windpipe is called the Heimlich Maneuver. It was developed by Henry Heimlich, M.D., Professor of Advance Clinical Sciences, Xavier University, Cincinnati, Ohio. The Maneuver works on the theory that the piece of food is like a cork in a bottle with air trapped below it. If you can squeeze the air out quickly it will force or pop the obstruction out. Even after a person exhales there is enough air left in the lungs to create air flow sufficient to dislodge the food. This method is explained under Home Treatment.

The important thing to remember before trying the Heimlich Maneuver is that it should be used on a choked victim. If the victim is coughing but still getting plenty of air, chances are the object isn't completely blocking the airway. If the coughing persists and the victim turns blue then proceed to use the Heimlich Maneuver. The Maneuver will be effective since it causes a flow of air, similar to the action of a bellows, that will carry the object out of the mouth. Also you need to make sure the victim is choked rather than having a heart attack. The 2 emergencies sometimes appear similar except for 1 big difference. The heart victim is usually breathing and complains of pain. The choked person cannot breathe or talk. Ask the victim if she or he can talk. If not, and other symptoms indicate a choked victim, use the Heimlich Maneuver.

PREVENTION

- Don't drink too much alcohol before eating. A person with dulled senses may not chew food properly and may try to swallow too large a portion of food.
- Don't eat and laugh at the same time. Food can be sucked into the windpipe.
- Take small bites. Cut meat into small pieces.
- Chew your food thoroughly.
- Don't give children under 5 years of age peanuts, popcorn, gum, or hard candy. They don't have molars developed yet and can't thoroughly chew these types of snacks. They can easily choke on these foods.

HOME TREATMENT

- Try the Heimlich Maneuver. You may have to use this maneuver several times before it is successful.
- If the victim is standing or sitting, follow the steps below.
  - o Wrap your arms around the victim's waist. If seated, reach around the back of the chair. You need to turn the person sideways if your arms won't reach around both victim and chair.
  - o Make a fist, put it into the palm of your other hand, and place the fist against the victim's abdomen above the navel and below the ribcage. Your fist should be thumb side against the abdomen.
  - o Apply a sudden upward pressure or thrust and the food should pop out. Repeat several times if necessary.
- If the victim is on the floor, follow the steps below. This position is also used where the rescuer is too small to reach around the victim. In this position, the weight of the rescuer can be used, rather than their strength. Children have saved their parents in this manner.

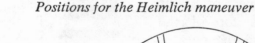

Positions for the Heimlich maneuver

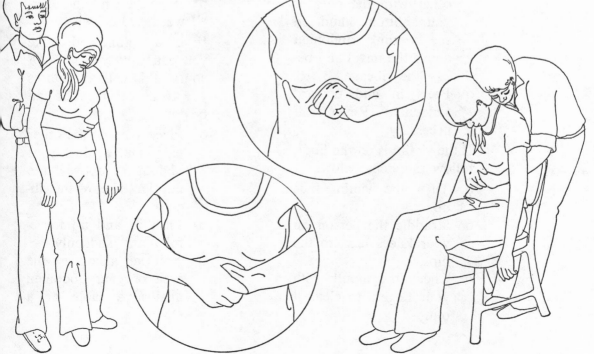

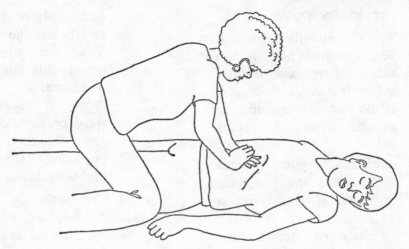

Heimlich maneuver for a horizontal victim

o Turn the victim face up.
o Straddle the person on your knees next to the hips.
o Place one of your hands on top of the other with the heel of your bottom hand on the victim's abdomen above the navel and below the ribcage.
o Press in and upward suddenly. Repeat if necessary.
• If the victim is on the floor, follow the steps below.
o Turn the victim face up.
o Straddle the person on your knees next to the hips.
o Check the mouth with your fingers to clear it out.

o Place one of your hands on top of the other with the heel of your hand on the victim's abdomen above the navel and below the ribcage.
o Press down and forward suddenly.
• If you are alone and choke you can save yourself. Of course, this method requires you to be calm but it can be done.
o Place 1 fist in the other palm and against your abdomen above the navel and below the ribcage.
o Push in and up forcefully and suddenly.
o You can also press the area of your abdomen against a table or a chair.

WHEN TO CALL A HEALTH PROFESSIONAL

- Call even if the food has been dislodged from a choked victim. There could be abdominal damage from the maneuver or the throat could be damaged by the object.

Emergency Room Usage

Hospital emergency rooms are staffed and equipped to offer sophisticated lifesaving services to those in need. They are designed and run to handle serious medical emergencies. Unfortunately many people use emergency departments for minor problems, which will cost them more than a visit to a physician's office and usually mean a longer wait for treatment.

Emergency departments are not set up to deal with minor illnesses. For example, they do not follow a first-come, first-served procedure. They take patients according to the severity of their illnesses. A cold, flu, or earache may have to wait for hours as a string of more critical problems are treated.

Emergency department services are also expensive because of the high cost of facilities and personnel needed. A family physician can treat an earache much more quickly and at a much lower cost. A family physician also keeps medical histories of each patient so possible allergies or drug interactions will be noted.

Try to rationally assess any illness or injury to determine if you can wait until the next day to see your health professional. However, if you feel you really do have an emergency and cannot reach your health professional, then do go to the emergency department for experienced help.

Heat Exhaustion

Heat exhaustion is also called heat prostration or heat collapse. It is a serious condition, caused by the loss of vital body fluids.

Anytime you work or play in hot weather you perspire. The perspiration evaporates and cools your skin. If you didn't perspire, your body would get hotter and hotter until you died. Perspiration is made up of water and salt. If your body is low on these elements and thus cannot perspire, heat exhaustion can occur.

Heat exhaustion does have warning signals. You may become dizzy, nauseated, or weak. You will appear pale and your skin will be cool and clammy. As soon as you feel any of these symptoms get out of the sun immediately and begin home treatment.

PREVENTION

- Avoid strenuous outdoor physical activity during the hottest part of the day.

- Wear light-colored clothing that reflects the sun's rays and is loose-fitting for better sweat evaporation.
- Try to avoid sudden changes of temperatures. Before getting into a car that's closed up and parked in the sun, open the doors and wait a few minutes. This is especially true if you just dashed out of an air-conditioned building.
- Drink plenty of water. You need to replace the fluids you are losing in sweat.
- Do not take salt tablets to prevent heat exhaustion. Your body usually loses more water than salt when you perspire so you need water rather than the salt.

HOME TREATMENT

- Get out of the sun to a cool spot.
- Drink lots of water.
- Eat salty foods such as crackers or salted nuts.
- If you are nauseous or dizzy, lie down awhile in a cool spot and then start taking water a little at a time.

WHEN TO CALL A HEALTH PROFESSIONAL

Heat exhaustion can sometimes lead to heat stroke. Although heat stroke is not common, it can be fatal if professional treatment isn't found. If you find any of the following symptoms, seek immediate help:

- The skin is dry, even under the arms.
- The temperature is high and keeps rising.
- The victim becomes unconscious.
- The skin is bright red.

While waiting for help to arrive start cooling the victim off. This can be done in a couple of ways:

- Remove the victim's clothes and sprinkle water over the body or apply wet, cold towels. Encourage evaporation by placing the victim in front of an air conditioner or by fanning him or her.
- Try rubbing ice cubes over the victim's arms and legs.

Hyperventilation

Hyperventilation is overbreathing or breathing too fast. Too much oxygen is taken in and the level of carbon dioxide is lowered in the blood. Hyperventilation is usually caused by anxiety and can also be a reaction to severe abdominal pain.

The victim of hyperventilation breathes fast and cannot seem to get enough air. Other symptoms include tingling or numbness of the skin around the mouth, feet, or hands. In severe cases there can be chest pain, spasms of the hand muscles, or even unconsciousness.

PREVENTION

- If you know someone has a history of hyperventilation and you notice fast breathing, bring it to the person's attention. In the final stages of hyperventilation victims may not be aware that they are breathing fast. After the initial stages victims are unable to control breathing voluntarily. So when you first notice it, try to get the person to only take a breath once every 5 seconds.

HOME TREATMENT

- The victim needs to increase the amount of carbon dioxide in the lungs. This can be done by breathing into a paper bag which covers the nose and mouth. Continue this treatment for 5–15 minutes.

WHEN TO CALL A HEALTH PROFESSIONAL

- If hyperventilation occurs in a person who doesn't appear tense or anxious. Sometimes, however, it can be difficult to determine if someone is tense or anxious. See Chapter 11, page 182 to help you determine if a person is anxious.

Hypothermia

Hypothermia is the lowering of the temperature of the body's inner core. It occurs whenever the body is losing more heat than it can produce. The air temperature, wind, and wetness all affect the rate at which heat leaves our bodies. Muscle activity such as exercise or even shivering burns up stored body fats to produce heat and warm the body. When the several cooling conditions combine as in a cold wet wind, the body's heat production methods are hard pressed to keep up with the heat loss. If heat loss continues, the body temperature will drop and hypothermia will set in.

Hypothermia can occur at outside temperatures as high as 45° F. Such cool weather with a damp wind can rob a poorly dressed person of heat in just a few hours. Extreme cold, especially with a wind can cause hypothermia much more quickly.

Early recognition is very important in the treatment of hypothermia. Often one hiker will lose heat to a very critical degree before others in the group notice anything wrong. If anyone begins to shiver violently, stumble, or will not coherently respond to questions, suspect hypothermia and warm that person up quickly.

PREVENTION

- Anytime you plan to be out-of-doors for several hours in cool or unsettled weather the following precautions should be taken:
  o Dress warmly and carry wind and waterproof clothing. Wool is the only fabric that is warm when wet.
  o Wear a warm hat. An unprotected head may lose up to one-half of the body's total heat production at 40° F.
  o Eat well before going out and carry extra food.
  o Head for shelter if you get wet or cold.
  o Don't drink alcohol while in the cold. It causes the body to lose heat faster.

HOME TREATMENT

- The best treatment is to put the victim in a tub of water at 110° F. Since this is not always available, try the methods below and maintain the warmth until help arrives.
  o Get the victim out of the wind and rain as best as is possible.

o Remove wet clothing and replace with dry or wool clothing if possible.
o Use body heat to warm the victim. Get inside a sleeping bag with the victim or wrap yourself in a blanket with the victim. If several people are with you, have everyone huddle around the victim.
o If the victim is conscious, administer warm fluids such as sweetened tea, broth, or juice. Have the victim eat candy and other quick energy foods.
o Do not give food or drink if the victim is unconscious.
o Do not give alcoholic beverages in any circumstance.

WHEN TO CALL A HEALTH PROFESSIONAL

- Get the victim to medical care as soon as possible if:
  o the victim seems confused. This is one of the first signs of hypothermia.
  o the body temperature does not return to normal.
  o the victim is a child or is elderly. It's a good idea to call regardless

of the severity of the symptoms.

Poisoning

Children will swallow just about anything, including poisonous substances. When in doubt of a poisoning, assume the worst. Always believe a child who indicates that some poison has been swallowed no matter how unappetizing the substance may seem to you. You will not harm anyone who has not swallowed poison by following the steps in Home Treatment.

If you suspect food poisoning, see page 34.

PREVENTION

About 80% of childhood poisonings occur to children aged 1–4. Infants grow so fast that sometimes they are crawling, walking children before we have had time to prepare to protect them. Develop habits of poison prevention before your child is born and certainly before she or he is crawling.

All drugs need to be locked from curious children. This includes aspirin. The most common source of childhood poisoning is aspirin, especially the chewable, flavored baby aspirin. No matter how often you give a dose of a drug, lock up that drug between doses.

Check under your kitchen sink for any poisons such as drain opener, dishwasher detergent, oven cleaner, or plant food. Remove poisons and put them completely out of reach of children. Dishwasher detergent is an especially dangerous substance. As more families each year enjoy the convenience of a dishwasher, more children die from the caustic poison of the detergent.

Always use original containers. Children recognize shapes and colors rather than labels. If you put plant food in a pop bottle, a child will think the bottle contains pop and may drink it.

If you cannot remove the under-the-sink poisons because of convenience or lack of room elsewhere, check into childproof latches for your cupboards. These plastic latches can be purchased at a hardware store and are installed in each cupboard with just a couple of screws. They are designed so adult fingers can reach and release the latch but short child fingers cannot. These latches are especially useful for cupboards with magnetic or "touch" releases.

HOME TREATMENT

- Give the poisoned victim a glass of milk. This will dilute poisons that shouldn't be vomited and will do no harm if the poison should be vomited.
- Call a Poison Control Center, hospital, or health professional to learn treatment for specific products

and to determine if it is safe to induce vomiting. Do *not* have the victim vomit if she or he:

o is having convulsions

o is unconscious

o has a burning sensation in the mouth or throat

o is known to have swallowed a corrosive agent or a petroleum product. Examples of such products include dishwasher detergent, lye, bleach, disinfectants, drain openers, floor wax, kerosene, or grease removers.

o Call a health professional immediately if any of these conditions are present.

• Induce vomiting if none of the above is evident. Syrup of ipecac is an effective way to start the vomiting and should be kept in every home where small children live or visit. See page 219 for a discussion of syrup of ipecac. If you don't have this essential drug, induce vomiting by placing your finger or a spoon in the back of the victim's throat.

• When vomiting begins, place the victim with head lower than the chest to prevent the vomited material from entering the lungs.

WHEN TO CALL A HEALTH PROFESSIONAL

• Whenever a poisoning is suspected. Call a health professional even if you have induced vomiting.

Seat Restraints

In 1975, 45,000 deaths occurred on American highways. Probably ⅔ of these accidents were humanly preventable. If you die between 15–35 years of age, an accident will be the likely cause of your death. Seat restraints save lives and minimize injuries.

There are 4 types of seat restraints, each with a distinct purpose. The 4 are infant carriers, child seats, seat belts, and lap-shoulder belts.

INFANT CARRIERS

Some new parents spend more time deciding what type of diaper to buy than they do finding a safe infant carrier to protect the new baby. Purchase a proper carrier before the baby is born and always use the carrier. In a crash your arms cannot prevent a child from going through a windshield. Even in an ordinary sudden stop, a child's forward momentum can be more than you have strength to stop.

Buy an infant carrier that is designed to be fastened in place by your car's seat belts. Some infant carriers can be converted into child seats as your baby grows. Such planning may help you justify a quality restraint that will protect your child if an accident occurs.

The carrier you buy should have good padding around the head and shoulders. A restraint that has an impact shield rather than a harness is safer. Most infant carriers will be safer if they are placed in the back seat facing backwards. Infants started in this position become accustomed to it.

Infants can ride in a carrier until they weigh 15 pounds and can hold their heads up. At that time you'll need to convert the carrier to a child seat or buy a child seat if yours does not convert.

CHILD SEATS

Child seats are fastened in a car by seat belts or by anchoring the seat to the car. The type that needs to be anchored has a strap that fastens to the shelf behind the back seat. Before buying such a restraint be sure the shelf in your car is made of metal rather than cardboard.

Again, look for good padding around the head and shoulders. A safety shield, a curved plastic shell which is fitted in front of the child, provides better protection. But if you cannot keep your child in the seat because of the shield, a harness type is better. The harness type usually allows a child to see more easily.

You will probably be able to put your child in a car seat with less fuss if the child was accustomed to an infant carrier. The child might also use seat belts more readily. It has also been found that children who use car seats are better behaved in a car than those who don't.

Children usually outgrow child seats when they reach a weight of about 30 pounds. They should then start using seat belts.

SEAT BELTS

Children under 4½ feet tall who weigh more than 30 pounds need to use a seat belt only. If they are under 4½ feet tall, a shoulder strap should not be used because it can cause serious damage to the neck in an accident. If your car has the lap and shoulder belts combined, place the child in the seat, latch the belt, and then have the child wiggle the body out of the shoulder restraint. The child should now be seated with the shoulder restraint behind the back.

If your child complains about not being able to see out the window, try to find a booster chair. The seat belt should go through the chair then around the child. This way the child and seat will be held in place in case of a sudden stop.

Shock

Shock occurs when vital tissues of the body do not get enough blood. It is usually present after severe injuries because of blood loss to the injured area. The leak in the circulatory system causes the blood pressure to drop below that needed to push blood to the brain and other organs.

Shock can also occur when the injury appears minor and insignificant. In such cases the body is so stunned by the injury that it loses control of the circulatory system. The blood vessels relax and expand instead of pushing the blood on through. Again, the blood pressure drops and vital organs are deprived of their needed blood supply. This condition can also occur when there has been no injury at all such as when a person is emotionally "shocked" by bad news. Common fainting is very similar to such shock, but a person quickly recovers from fainting.

The symptoms of shock are the same regardless of the cause. They include cold and clammy skin, a fast, weak pulse that increases in rate, lowering blood pressure, paleness in the face, dizziness, nausea, and dilated pupils. Restlessness and anxiety often precede or accompany other symptoms. As shock progresses, the victim may slur his or her speech.

Shock must be considered a serious threat to life. The longer a person is allowed to worsen, the greater the danger. Prompt action may well save the victim's life.

PREVENTION

Since shock can occur any time there is an injury or serious emotional shock, preventive measures should be started even before symptoms appear. The steps under Home Treatment should be followed.

HOME TREATMENT

- Have the victim lie down.
- Elevate the legs 2 inches or more off the ground. If injury is to the head or chest, keep the legs flat.
- Treat all injuries and splint fractures. See Splinting, page 140.
- Keep the victim warm, but not hot. Place a blanket under the victim and cover with sheet or blanket depending on the weather.
- Allow the victim to drink small amounts of water unless there is possible abdominal injury, vomiting, or unconsciousness.
- Take and record the victim's pulse every 5 minutes.
- Comfort and reassure the victim to relieve anxiety.

WHEN TO CALL A HEALTH PROFESSIONAL

- Anyone with significant symptoms of shock should be evaluated by a health professional as soon as possible. These symptoms are:
  o cold and clammy skin
  o fast, weak pulse or a pulse which increases in rate

    o low blood pressure
    o paleness in the face
    o dizziness
    o nausea
    o dilated pupils
    o slurring of speech

Spinal Injury

Any accident involving the neck or back must be considered a possible spinal injury. Permanent paralysis may be avoided if the victim is immobilized and moved correctly.

Symptoms of a spinal injury are pain, bruises on the head, neck, shoulders, or back area, increased pain with the slightest movement, loss of sensation or movement in hands, feet, arms, or legs, a "tingly" feeling in the limbs, weakness or numbness on 1 side of the body, or tenderness at 1 point along the neck.

HOME TREATMENT

- If you suspect a spinal injury do not move the person unless there is an immediate threat to life, such as fire. Don't drag victims from automobile wrecks. If the injury was a diving accident, float the person face up in the water until skilled medical help arrives. The water will act as a splint and keep the spinal column immobile. Don't pull the victim from the water as you may cause permanent damage.

- Seek medical help to transport the person.

WHEN TO CALL A HEALTH PROFESSIONAL

- Whenever a spinal injury is suspected.

Suicide

Many people have considered suicide at some time in their lives as a possible escape from a crisis. Fortunately, it is usually a passing thought that isn't acted upon. However, when a casual thought changes to intention, then to an actual plan, the threats of physical harm or death greatly increase. A person planning a suicide can give you signals ranging from telling you that they feel worthless, (which may be the only signal you will be given), to giving you the details of the suicide plan. Always take these signals a person gives seriously. Using your common sense and a direct communication approach, you can usually determine if the suicide risk is great. If it is, your appropriate action might save a life.

Suicidal people are usually in the midst of a crisis. Faced with a problem that has overwhelming importance to them, they may not see any alternative but suicide. Since these people have conflicting feelings of wanting to live and wanting to die, you may have a good chance of preventing suicide. They are asking for help by telling you their intentions of suicide, so you have a chance to act.

PREVENTION

- Generally, establish an open and direct relationship to find out whether the person has a suicide plan and what it is. "How are you going to do it?" "Have you decided when?" Do not be afraid to talk specifically about their ideas regarding death. They have informed you of the plans, so try to matter-of-factly speak to them without undue anxiety. This will be helpful in reducing the person's own anxiety about the suicide. You must also be the judge of how lethal the proposed plan is. Is the method really deadly? Using a gun, jumping out of a window, driving while drunk? Is the means available? Does the person have specific plans as to when and where?
- You may be able to help the person by finding out what exactly was the cause of the crisis. Help the person reconstruct the chain of events that led to the crisis. For some people just talking and realizing that a particular event led to their anxiety is enough for them to become less anxious.

- Finally, arrange for yourself, a close friend, or relative to be with the person for that day or night to show concern and offer support. During the suicidal crisis the person is depending on you for help. You can help them and may prevent their death, if you are sensitive to their feelings, direct in your discussions, and not overly anxious.

WHEN TO CALL A HEALTH PROFESSIONAL

- If a person indicates that adequate preparations have been made for the suicide, then the potential danger is great and you need to seek professional help immediately.
- If you have any questions or doubts of the suicidal risk of a person, refer them to a mental health professional for an in-depth evaluation. If the person resists seeing someone, then use the resource yourself. You could share your own anxiety and responsibility and have a professional clarify the risk of danger and offer alternative solutions. If you are unsure whom to contact, call a community mental health center, suicide prevention center, hot-

line, hospital emergency room, or clinic.

Unconsciousness

An unconscious person is completely unaware of what is going on and is unable to make purposeful movements. Fainting is a form of brief unconsciousness while a coma is a deep, prolonged state of unconsciousness.

Causes of unconsciousness include stroke, epilepsy, fainting, heat exhaustion, diabetic coma, insulin shock, head injury, suffocation, drunkenness, shock, bleeding and heart attack.

HOME TREATMENT

- It is important that the unconscious person can breathe sufficiently. Check for breathing and if necessary, open the airway and begin artificial respiration. See page 143 for how to do these procedures.
- Check the pulse. If there is none, start cardiopulmonary resuscitation (CPR). See CPR, page 146.
- Treat any injuries.
- Keep the victim lying down.
- Do not give the victim anything by mouth.
- Look for medical identification. The victim may have a bracelet, necklace, or card that identifies the medical problem such as epilepsy, diabetes, or allergy to certain drugs.
- If you find that the victim is a diabetic, he or she may have insulin shock (insufficient sugar in the blood) or be in a diabetic coma (too much sugar in the blood). The symptoms of a diabetic coma are red, dry skin; weak, rapid pulse; and gasping for air. Symptoms of insulin shock are pale, moist skin, normal pulse, and shallow breathing. If the person is a known diabetic and starts to lose consciousness, give something sweet to eat or drink. This will help if they are experiencing insulin shock and won't hurt if they are going into a coma. Remember, though, do not give anything to an unconscious person.

WHEN TO CALL A HEALTH PROFESSIONAL

- A victim of a head injury needs to be carefully observed. See Head Injuries, page 134. See a health professional if the person loses consciousness after the injury.
- Unconscious victims always need to be seen by a health professional.

9

Dental Care

The goal of good dental care is to keep your natural teeth all your life. It's a goal that almost anyone can achieve.

Dental disease is an optional health problem. Your family can choose not to have it. With good home care you just don't have to lose your teeth.

Plaque and Tooth Decay

Bacteria are always present in the mouth. When well-fed and undisturbed they attach themselves to the teeth and multiply into larger and larger bacterial colonies called plaque. These masses of germs appear as a sticky but colorless film on your teeth.

This sticky plaque does 2 unfortunate things. First, food particles, especially refined sugars, stick to it. It uses that food to grow more bacteria and to produce acid. You wouldn't think that a little acid, even from a million germs, could eat through tooth enamel, especially with all that saliva in the mouth to dilute it. It couldn't—*if* it were diluted. That's where the sticky plaque comes in again. It holds the acids against the tooth surface and prevents the saliva from mixing with it. Even swishing with water can't get to the acid under its sticky blanket of plaque.

Fortunately, it takes about 24 hours for enough bacteria and acid to build up to do damage to your teeth, enough time for you to get the plaque off your teeth and to wash away the acid. But if you eat a lot of sugar, especially between-meal sugary snacks such as candy, cake, or chewing gum, plaque can build up incredibly fast. Then cleaning the plaque and acid off your teeth may be required more frequently.

Plaque and Gum Disease

Bacterial plaque is also the cause of gum disease. Again, the toxins and acids damage the healthy layers of skin that touch the teeth right at the gum line. The skin of your gums is similar to any other part of your skin. When it's healthy, it's a strong, tough layer that protects what's inside. But when it's irritated, it becomes tender and is likely to bleed. Gums which bleed frequently are a definite sign of gum disease.

As the disease progresses, more and more the skin and fibers that fasten the gums to the teeth are destroyed. The gums then pull away from the teeth leaving deepening pockets between the gums and teeth which are perfect breeding grounds for more bacteria to form and damage the newly exposed portions of the teeth and gums. Eventually, the gum attachments can be destroyed all the way down to the jaw bone that supports the teeth. The teeth then get looser and looser.

Calculus or dental tartar is also caused by plaque. Actually, tartar is formed from mineral deposits which get trapped by the plaque and are eventually deposited on the tooth. Once this happens, professional help is usually needed to remove it. Although the tartar itself is not the cause of gum disease, it does prevent the gum line from being cleaned of plaque through regular brushing and flossing and so indirectly contributes to the problem. Of course, if the plaque is regularly removed in the first place, there will be much less opportunity for the tartar to form.

Do You Have Gum Disease?

If your gums bleed, you probably have gum disease. How easily and frequently they bleed is a good measure of both how diseased they are and how long it will take to get them healthy again.

If your gums bleed when you push on them or bleed often when you brush your teeth—that's bad. If they only bleed once in a while on the dental floss, it's not good but it won't take as long to get back to the healthy gum stage. Either way, proper home care should show significant improvements in just a few weeks. And either way, the time to start is *now!*

How to Brush

Brushing should remove dental plaque from the outer, inner, and chewing surfaces of the teeth. A *soft-bristle* toothbrush is most effective in removing the plaque. Ideally, each bristle should be rounded at the tip. Having a good brush is very important but it's what you do with it that really makes the difference. The following method of brushing is one that is recommended for effective tooth care:

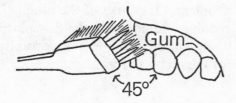

Brush at a 45° angle

1. Place the brush at a 45° angle where the teeth meet the gums. Press firmly, and gently wiggle or rock the brush back and forth using small circular movements. Do not scrub if you have a stiff-bristle brush. Vigorous brushing can cause the gums to recede and the teeth to show abrasion.
2. Brush all surfaces of the teeth—tongue-side and cheek-side. Give special attention to the front teeth and behind the back teeth since they are the most often overlooked.
3. Brush the chewing surfaces vigorously with short back and forth strokes.
4. Brush the tongue. Plaque on the tongue can cause bad breath and is a nursery for bacterial growth.
5. Use disclosing tablets periodically to see if any plaque is being left on the teeth.

Note: Brushing with just water is often more effective than using toothpaste since the brusher can better see and feel what he or she is doing. If a toothpaste is used, a fluoride toothpaste is preferred.

DISCLOSING TABLETS

How well do you clean your teeth? You should be removing all the dental plaque from every tooth at least once a day. Unfortunately, it's hard to tell how well you are doing by just looking in the mirror. Plaque is a *colorless* film, remember.

Disclosing tablets are small, chewable tablets that help you see plaque. Chew the tablet, then swish with water. The tablets will color any plaque that remains on your teeth. By using a flashlight and a dental mirror you can see for yourself where you or your children have been missing the plaque. Any plaque spots you see on the teeth may be sites for decay. Also, any spots around the gum line could signal the beginning of gum disease.

Disclosing tablets are not expensive and can be found at most drugstores. Once you properly clean your teeth, they leave no stain or trace of color. These tablets provide the immediate feedback you and your children need to develop good home care habits. Adults should use tablets as they think necessary. Children should use them at least once per month to reinforce good brushing habits.

DENTAL FLOSSING

Daily flossing is the best single way to prevent gum disease and dental decay between the teeth. Unfortunately, most people either have never learned how to floss or have never figured out how to make it part of their daily routine.

Many people believe the only purpose of flossing is to remove particles of food that get caught between the teeth. Not so. The real purpose of flossing is to scrape off the dental plaque which forms between the teeth and just under the gum line. Those places are usually impossible to clean adequately by brushing alone.

Flossing cleans the plaque off the surfaces of the teeth and allows the saliva to neutralize and wash away the acids and other irritants.

Flossing does require some dexterity and a little practice. It should be done once a day at a regular time. After learning to floss in front of a mirror a person should try flossing without one. That will make it a lot easier to fit flossing into a regular daily routine. For example, many people floss while watching television or while soaking in the tub.

There are many different kinds of dental floss on the market today: waxed floss, unwaxed floss, extra fine floss, flossing tape, and flossing ribbons. Each has its own advantages. Each person should select the type that works best on his or her teeth.

HOW TO FLOSS

There are a number of effective ways to hold the dental floss. Following is a description of 2 methods:

1. The finger-wrap method: Cut off a piece of floss 18–20 inches long. Pinch the end of the floss between the left thumb and the middle of the left middle finger. Wrap the floss around the finger several times and repeat this procedure on the right hand, until the 2 hands are a thumb-length apart.

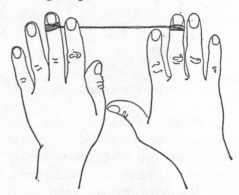

Wrapping dental floss

2. The circle method: Cut off a piece of floss 12 inches long. Tie the ends together to form a loop about the size of an orange. If the loop is too large, wrap the floss around the middle fingers to make it smaller.

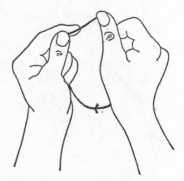

Flossing the upper teeth

For the upper teeth use a thumb of one hand and forefinger of the other as shown in the figure.

For the lower teeth use both forefingers to guide the floss, the fingers should be close together (about ½ inch apart).

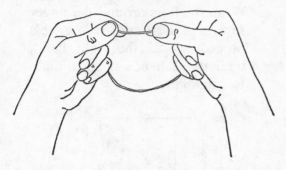

Flossing the lower teeth

A variety of flossing tools are available for those who prefer them. They are particularly handy when an adult flosses a child's teeth since it's hard to get adult-sized fingers in a child-sized mouth. Many adults find them equally helpful for their own teeth. Flossing tools can do a good job of cleaning if care is taken to curve the floss around the tooth and partly under the gum line. Again, it is the scraping action that yields the benefits.

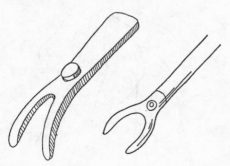

Flossing tools

The most important thing about flossing is to curve the floss around the tooth being cleaned and to gently slide the floss under the gum line. With both fingers holding the floss firmly against the tooth, move floss up and down several times to scrape the plaque off. Often the teeth will sound "squeaky clean." Popping the floss in and out without using the scraping action will not remove much plaque.

At first flossing may be awkward and slow, but continued practice will increase skill and effectiveness. Any bleeding should subside as the gums become healthy.

Home Care for Children

Efforts to save your children's teeth should start long before their permanent teeth arrive. In fact, dental care really starts in pregnancy. A baby's first teeth begin to form before birth. Good nutrition in the mother is very important.

From birth on, the child begins to develop life-long habits of dental care. If a small child's mouth is kept clean even before the teeth arrive, the feel of a clean mouth may encourage good habits as the child grows. Infants and small children should not be given bottles of fruit juice, jello water, or even milk to go to sleep with or to constantly suck on. Such constant contact between the young teeth and the sugar in the liquids can cause rapid dental decay. Toothbrushing should begin when the first teeth come in. Then for the next 4–5 years the parents must take the responsibility of brushing the child's teeth. Only after children develop enough dexterity to tie their own shoelaces, should they take over the entire brushing routine. Even then, use disclosing tablets often to determine if a child is able to remove all of the plaque. A good training method is to have the child brush in the morning and the parent at night until the art of brushing is mastered. Then, a once a day routine can be started.

Parents should try brushing their children's teeth both with and without toothpaste. A fluoride toothpaste may help strengthen the tooth surfaces, but brushing with just water will help you better see what you are doing.

Flossing, too, should be started by the parents of a child as soon as the child has teeth that touch each other. Flossing tools may be particularly helpful in doing a good job in a small mouth. A child cannot usually take over the flossing job until around age 8. The actual timing depends a lot on the child's dexterity and motor skills.

Brushing and flossing provide a special opportunity for parents and children to feel close to each other. Try to look on it not as drudgery but as an expression of love. Don't confine the activity to a bathroom. Find a comfortable spot for all concerned. One easy way is to sit on a couch and have the child sit on the floor in front of you resting the neck and head on the couch between your knees.

During brushing and flossing your children are a captive and usually willing audience. Use the moment to teach about self-care of their own bodies.

Professional Dental Care for Children

Every child should visit the dentist early in life (before age 4). This first visit should get the child thinking positively about dentistry. It is usually a quick, inexpensive check-up and get-to-know-you session with a little dental education thrown in. It may save a lot of anxiety later. Subsequent visits might include a more thorough examination with or without dental X-rays.

After that, even if all is well, your dentist will probably recommend 6-month check-ups. Since many of us do not take proper care of our teeth, a check-up every 6 months is not too frequent. On the other hand, if you and your child *do* take good care of your teeth and have had a few perfect check-ups in a row, ask your dentist if less frequent appointments might be adequate.

How to Choose a Dentist

Most dentists are competent professionals capable of high quality dental care. Although all dentists recognize the importance of home brushing and flossing to dental care, many have low expectations of the amount of care their patients are willing to do. Consequently, many dentists resign themselves to repairing the continual damage done to the teeth by improper care. You may have to show your dentist that you are serious about saving your teeth if you want a full range of support and dental education as part of the professional services you receive.

If you have a choice of dentists in your area, select one who really believes in self-care. Any dentist who offers dental education as a part of each dental visit is obviously serious about helping you keep your teeth.

You can use your phone in your search for a preventively-oriented dentist, since it is a lot easier than visiting several offices. Call up the dentist's office and ask some questions. The answers should tell you how the dentist feels about the importance of saving your teeth. Ask what the initial visit to the dentist consists of. A thorough exam will include a medical history, a full mouth series of X-rays, a check of the gums as well as the teeth, an oral cancer exam, and an evaluation of the straightness and placement of the teeth in the mouth. Ask about fee arrangements. You should know the cost of treatment *before* it is begun. Most importantly, ask if the dentist has a regular prevention program to teach and reinforce your family in good dental care.

Once you find a winner, stick with your selection. You will invest a lot of money in your X-rays, dental records, and your dentist's own knowledge of you and your teeth. Switching will usually cause much duplication and unnecessary expense. If you must change, try to get the old dentist to give you your dental records or to send them to the new dentist.

Preventive Orthodontics

Orthodontics is a specialty in dentistry which deals with the straightening of teeth. Most people equate orthodontics with wearing braces so that teeth will look pretty, but there is more to it than that. Healthy teeth require contact with other teeth if they are to stay healthy. Therefore, poorly arranged teeth not only affect appearance but also influence the life and usefulness of the teeth.

Sometimes pending orthodontic trouble can be spotted early, while the baby teeth are still in the child's mouth. Preventive treatment then can often reduce or eliminate the need for braces later.

Dental X-rays are often effective in finding orthodontic trouble early. It's another of the many good reasons why professional dental check-ups should start early in a child's life.

10

Eating Wisely

Anyone who tries to grow houseplants knows you can't raise a healthy plant without the proper nutrients. The right amount of water and fertilizer at the right times makes all the difference in the life and health of a plant.

Our bodies also need the right nutrients in order to be healthy. Fortunately, the human body is more adaptable than a plant and adults can survive on a poor diet for a longer time. But most of us want to do more than just survive. We want to thrive. Good eating habits can help you do just that. The right fuel keeps our bodies operating at their best each day, and helps us ward off illness and recover from crises such as surgery or severe physical or mental stress.

More and more medical evidence indicates that the way we eat can affect the length of our lives and may be a factor in some diseases. The American lifestyle, eating too much rich, fat food, too fast, may be harmful to our health.

As adults our eating habits are deeply ingrained, and it is difficult but not impossible to change them once you decide it's worth some effort. Obviously, it's easier to start out with good habits. Therefore, this chapter gives some guidelines to good eating and some hints on how to help your children establish healthy eating habits. The best way children learn is by example so you can help them most by practicing good nutrition along with them.

Obesity—A Large Problem

Eating well doesn't mean eating a lot, but unfortunately, too many of us believe it does. Obesity is a major health problem in the United States today.

Insurance companies have estimated that for each pound in excess of 10 pounds overweight, a person loses 1 month of life. It doesn't take much to cut a whole year from your life. There are also indications that the obese person has a tendency to high blood pressure, heart disease, and diabetes.

Am I overweight? That's pretty easy to answer when you're honest with yourself. Determining what your ideal weight should be is a little trickier. One guess would be what you weighed at age 25, if you weren't then overweight.

Weight charts, such as the one from the U. S. Department of Agriculture reproduced on page 174, can serve as rough guides to ideal weight. The low, average, and high weights for each height correspond roughly to frame size. If you feel you have a small frame, consider the average weight as a maximum for you, and so on.

Weight charts have a limited value, however, because they cannot take into account the amount of body fat you carry. And excess body fat, not just excess weight, is the hazard to your health.

The best test for excess body fat is an honest appraisal in front of a mirror. That extra roll at the waistline probably isn't muscle. If you're still not convinced, take the "pinch test." Pull out and pinch the skin on the bottom of your upper arm between your thumb and forefinger. If there is a thickness of an inch or more between your thumb and finger, chances are you're carrying excess fat. (This test is most meaningful for persons under 50 years of age.)

Weight control is a challenge, but it can be done. To maintain your weight, you balance the calories you consume against those your body uses each day. To lose weight, you must use more calories each day than you consume. This causes the body to use calories which had been stored as fat, and thus you lose weight. So a 125 pound woman needs about 1,500 calories a day to maintain her weight. If she consumes fewer calories, or burns more through added activity, she will lose weight. It's obvious that the amount of calories you need each day varies greatly according to individual needs and activity levels. As you grow older, basal metabolism (the rate the resting body burns food to perform necessary life functions) slows, so older people need fewer calories, but the same amount of nutrients. Although this sounds relatively simple, other factors make it more complicated.

It is impractical, if not impossi-

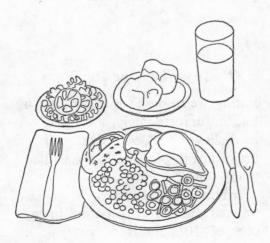

ble, to accurately count all the calories you consume daily, but calories do count. By eating just 100 calories more than you need each day, you can gain about 10 pounds in only 1 year. (That's 1 piece of buttered toast a day!) Here is where the balancing act comes in. To control weight, you must either decrease the calories you eat or increase the calories you burn through physical activity to maintain the balance. One pound of stored body fat equals 3,500 calories. To lose one pound per week, you would need to eat 500 calories less each day.

Obesity in children is especially troubling for three reasons. First, an obese child is more likely to be an obese adult. Eating habits are hard to unlearn, and change during adulthood is very difficult. Second, obesity in children can cause psychological problems. Heavy children may have difficulty participating in usual childhood games and activities. Teasing by playmates may cause them to participate less and less in physical activities. Sometimes this withdrawal leads to withdrawal from other social events. Third, as a reaction to a lack of peer acceptance, the overweight child may turn to more eating and gain satisfaction through food. It is difficult for these people to lose weight later because of the psychological comfort gained from eating.

Any efforts you might make early to avoid weight problems from developing in your child would be well worth it. Should your efforts fail to accomplish changes, or if your child is already overweight, consider getting help from a health professional.

There are probably as many hints on weight control as there are pounds to lose. A few of the most sensible are:

- Don't worry constantly about weight. *That's* not good for you either.
- Take off extra pounds when you notice them. It's easier to take off 4 pounds now than 14 next year.
- Eat sensibly. Eat a variety of foods in reasonable amounts and cut down on extras such as soft drinks and desserts.
- If you must snack, make it a low calorie snack.
- Reduce the amount of fat in your diet. Eat lean meats and limit added fat from sources such as salad dressings, butter, margarine, and oils. Fats have the highest concentration of calories of any food.
- Serve small meals, on small plates, as attractively as you can.
- Do not crash diet. The rapid loss of several pounds almost inevitably followed by their gain back, repeated diet after diet, can be harmful. If you must lose large amounts, talk to a health

Approximate Desirable Weights

MEN

Height (without shoes)	Weight in pounds (without clothing)		
	Low*	Average*	High*
5'3"	118	129	141
5'4"	122	133	145
5'5"	126	137	149
5'6"	130	142	155
5'7"	134	147	161
5'8"	139	151	166
5'9"	143	155	170
5'10"	147	159	174
5'11"	150	163	178
6'0"	154	167	183
6'1"	158	171	188
6'2"	162	175	192
6'3"	165	178	195

WOMEN

	Low*	Average*	High*
5'0"	100	109	118
5'1"	104	112	121
5'2"	107	115	125
5'3"	110	118	128
5'4"	113	122	132
5'5"	116	125	135
5'6"	120	129	139
5'7"	123	132	142
5'8"	126	136	146
5'9"	130	140	151
5'10"	133	144	156
5'11"	137	148	161
6'0"	141	152	166

* Correspond roughly to small, medium and large frame.

professional about the safest way to do it.

- Get plenty of exercise. Moderate exercise should not increase your appetite, but rather help to better regulate it.

- Limit the amount of sugar you consume; you'll save pounds, teeth, and dollars.

- Watch your children's calorie balance. A child who is very active in summer may need less to eat in the winter when sitting in school for hours.

- Place enough food on your children's plates for a small helping and encourage them to sample everything. If they are still hungry, let them have a second small serving. When they are full, let them stop eating.

Starting Good Habits

Introducing a child to the world is fun, and teaching good eating habits can be part of that fun if you approach it right.

Once children leave home for part of the day, even if just for preschool or kindergarten, they start making food choices without their parents' guidance. If you start them from infancy with the right ideas about foods, they should make better choices when on their own.

Habits are learned. Even the "sweet tooth" is a learned habit. Parents who keep to a minimum the amount of sugar in their infants' and toddlers' diets are pleased to see their children choose fruit over candy—at least sometimes. It is easy to slip up and become lax about your child's eating patterns—but remember that you're helping your child establish the habits which will affect your child's health, well-being, and possibly even length of life.

Try to avoid giving food as a reward or withholding it as punishment. A child given an ice cream cone as a reward for good behavior or threatened with no dinner to curb bad behavior starts to look at food as something really special that must be earned. Then when the child feels the need of a reward or an ego booster, food seems the answer.

Offer your child a variety of foods but don't force the child to eat an unwanted food. A small taste and the observation of others eating is the best strategy in getting a child to try new foods. Imitation is a much better teacher than force. If you enjoy a food and are willing to try new ones, your child is more apt to do the same. Also, if you avoid having sugary, "junk" foods in the home, a child simply cannot eat them, at least at home.

Don't become overly concerned about your child's food intake. If you serve your family a wide variety of nutritious foods regularly and in a pleasant environment, you can relax and feel that you're providing the best "nutrition atmosphere" possible. Then, an occasional food "jag" of peanut butter sandwiches for breakfast, lunch, and dinner shouldn't worry you. Continue to offer and serve other foods without making it an issue and that food jag probably won't last long.

Remember, too, that each person is unique. Food likes and dislikes will vary in a family without harm, as long as good nutritional intake is kept up, and as long as no one expects to be constantly catered to.

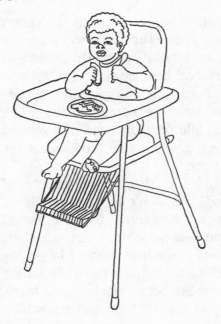

feel eating at an adult-sized table, in an adult chair. Booster seats or cushions, foot-stools, or simply chairs with high rungs can help equalize things. Child-sized utensils can be used too, if your child has trouble holding larger ones. And don't insist that your child hold utensils the way an adult does. Dexterity comes with age and the skill will improve with the desire to look like everyone else. In fact, don't fuss about utensils—fingers are fine until a child can hold utensils easily.

Just as a child's legs are shorter than an adult's, so is a child's stomach smaller. A small plate with small servings is a good idea. Let the child ask for seconds. It will make the child and the cook feel better. Because of their smaller storage capacities coupled with high calorie needs for size, children may need snacks to supplement meals. These snacks should provide part of the child's daily nutrient needs, and should not be served so close to a meal that they interfere with the child's mealtime appetite.

Physical and Emotional Environment

The physical and emotional environment at mealtimes has a profound effect on how we feel about food and eating.

Any serious weight watcher knows that a tiny meal on a small but pretty plate, attractively arranged and served, is more apt to satisfy the appetite than those same few morsels eaten standing in the kitchen. When children are served meals in a pleasant environment, they enjoy the eating experience, and may be more willing to try a variety of foods.

CHILD-SIZED ENVIRONMENT

Imagine yourself eating at a giant's table. That's how a child can

EMOTIONAL ENVIRONMENT

Ideally, mealtimes should be pleasant family experiences, time for good conversation and relaxation. However, for today's busy families dinner is often the only time the family is together and frequently that meal is made unpleasant by arguments or too much noise.

Try to make meals as pleasant as possible by keeping conversation pleasant, instead of a daily report of everyone's problems. Having the television on makes conversation difficult and causes people to ignore what and how much they're eating. Hardest of all, try to keep comments about your child's eating to a minimum.

Their meal and yours will be more pleasant. Anxiety about whether the child is getting enough to eat or making sure a child cleans the plate may inadvertently cause obesity. Children should be allowed to eat what they feel they need.

Healthy Snacks

Look on between-meal snacks as part of the day's total food intake, and be sure the snacks contribute more than "empty calories." This is especially important in a preschooler's diet, because of the high nutrient need in relation to calorie need.

Fruits and fruit juices are good snacks as are chunks of cheese, meat, or a cup of soup. Carrot and celery sticks, raw zucchini, or green pepper all taste good and are nutritious. When you want to give cookies or other sweets, be sure they contain more than just sugar. Oatmeal raisin cookies or carrot raisin cake are good substitutes for gooey pastries. The following recipe for Iron-Rich Cookies makes an excellent snack.

How to Recognize an Adequate Diet

Good nutrition means eating the food that will keep your body running at its peak. Although it's neither difficult nor expensive to get an adequate diet, many Americans, at all socio-economic levels, do not practice good nutrition. One major nutrition problem in America is obesity—many of us are simply

---

Iron-Rich Cookies

Cream 1½ cups brown sugar with ¾ cup margarine and add 2 slightly beaten eggs. Sift together ½ cup flour, 1 teaspoon soda, ½ teaspoon EACH salt, cinnamon, cloves and nutmeg. Flour 1 cup of raisins with part of this mixture. Add dry ingredients to the creamed mixture alternately with ½ cup milk. Then add 4 cups Baby Oatmeal, then the raisins.

Drop by heaping teaspoonfuls on greased baking sheet. Bake 10–12 minutes at 400°.

---

overnourished. Others need just a little guidance and thought to assure getting the foods to keep us healthiest.

The following sections give facts to help you provide your family with an adequate diet. Use them, then try not to worry if it appears your children "aren't eating enough to keep a bird alive." Unless your child is no growing, is continually listless, has pale skin, poor color, or has no appetite (refuses food for several days) try not to worry. If any of these signs occur, talk it over with a health professional.

Vitamins

Severe vitamin deficiency is rarely a problem in the United States today. The wide variety of foods available and modern preservation and packaging techniques, assure most of us an adequate intake of vitamins, if we choose from that wide variety of available foods. With the exceptions of pregnant and nursing women and infants, most people need not take vitamin supplements. At any rate, vitamin supplements will not make up for an inadequate diet. The whole diet must be con-

Foods Rich in Iron

Raisins	Whole grains	*Liver
Prunes	Dark green leafy	Red meats
Dried apricots	vegetables	*Oysters,
Iron-enriched	Dried peas	sardines,
cereals	and beans	shrimp

*These foods, particularly liver, are good sources of iron, but are also very high in cholesterol. This should be considered when selecting foods.

Iron

Inadequate iron intake can pose a problem for preschoolers and women, for it can lead to iron-deficiency anemia. Above is a list of foods which are good sources of iron. Regularly including these foods in the diet will help prevent iron deficiency. If anemia is suspected, a health professional can diagnose it by taking a blood test and may suggest iron supplements be used along with a diet high in iron to correct the problem.

sidered, as vitamins are only one of the many necessary nutrients. Vitamin or mineral supplements may be suggested by a health professional for a specific deficiency, but otherwise they are generally merely costly and unnecessary. More information on vitamins is in "Your Medicine Chest" on page 228.

Salt

Our diets don't need a lot of added salt. The amount used in cooking provides enough for our bodies' needs. Some families simply choose to keep the salt shaker off the dining table. Research suggests that continued overuse of salt may contribute to health problems such as hypertension and heart disease.

Sugar

The problem of too much sugar in our diets is a sticky one. The average American consumes about 130 pounds of sugar each year. That's almost 500 calories per person per day from sugar alone. Can we stand that? The high incidence of obesity and dental disease suggest not. One way to eliminate unneeded extra sugar is to avoid sugar-coated cereals. Some of these are up to 40–50% sugar. Read the box label. Ingredients are listed in descending order of amounts in the product. If sugar is listed first it means there's more sugar than cereal by weight in the box. Eating fresh fruits instead of canned is another way to avoid excess sugar, and raisins or nuts are good substitutes for candy.

Another way to decrease sugar intake is to cut down on high sugar foods such as sweetened beverages, candies, cakes, and pies in your diet.

Diet and Disease

There's a lot of talk today about the role of diet in the development of diseases, particularly of the heart and blood vessels. It's an area where much research is being conducted.

In the study of heart disease several factors have been identified which seem to increase the risk of disease. Smoking is a powerful factor. Heredity—the history of heart disease in your family—has a big effect on your chances of getting heart disease. Persons with high blood pressure run a greater risk of heart disease. Being overweight is also a factor, and lack of exercise also seems to make people more likely to develop heart problems.

Stress is another "risk factor." The level of fat and cholesterol in the blood has also been associated with a higher likelihood of heart disease.

As these risk factors combine, the chances of developing heart disease increase.

Research to date has not found a definite link between diet and heart disease. What it has found so far indicates that a person who has some of the risk factors mentioned would be prudent to make some changes in diet to reduce the risk factors of elevated blood fats and cholesterol. Special diets are available for those at high risk of disease. A health professional can measure the amount of cholesterol in your blood and make recommended dietary changes. It is important to remember that cholesterol is a natural substance present in all our bodies, which we need to survive.

In some persons, however, the level in the blood may reach a high level which appears to increase the risk of heart disease. What hasn't been proven for sure is what effect dietary intake of cholesterol has on the level of cholesterol in the blood.

The average healthy person who does not have any risk factors probably need make no drastic dietary changes if the present diet is nutritious. Almost everyone could benefit from reducing their sugar intake, for sugar is a prime factor behind dental disease, diabetes, and obesity. And, since fats provide the highest concentration of calories of any food, a sensible re- duction of fat intake can help prevent obesity, as well as reduce the fat content in the blood. Two simple ways to reduce fat intake are to drink low fat milk and to trim fats off meat.

Reducing the ratio of saturated animal fats (those solid at room temperature) to polyunsaturated vegetable fats (liquid at room temperature) has also been shown to lower the level of fat in the blood.

Animal fats contain a lot of cholesterol, so reducing their intake will reduce cholesterol intake. If you choose to specifically avoid foods containing cholesterol, liver, eggs, and shrimp are the highest sources of cholesterol.

Basic Food Groups

Choosing a wide variety of foods from each of the food groups listed below will help your family get an adequate diet. Try to include lots of fresh fruits and vegetables.

FOOD GROUPS	MINIMUM DAILY FOOD NEEDS	
	ADULTS	PRESCHOOLERS
MEAT Lean meats, fish, poultry, eggs or meat alternates (dried beans, peas, nuts)	2 servings (3–4 ounce serving)	2 servings (2–3 ounce serving)
DAIRY PRODUCTS Milk (low-fat), cheese, etc.	2 servings (6–8 ounce serving)	3 servings (6–8 ounce serving)
VEGETABLES AND FRUITS Always include dark green or yellow vegetables, citrus fruits or tomatoes	4 or more servings (½ cup serving)	4 servings (⅓–½ cup serving)
BREADS AND CEREALS Wheat bread and whole grain cereals provide needed fiber and are preferable to white breads and pastries from highly refined flours. Avoid sugar coated cereals.	3 servings (1 slice bread or ¼–¾ cup cereal)	4 servings (½–1 slice bread or ¼–¾ cup cereal)

11

Mental Wellness

Good family self-care cannot ignore mental health. Our mental wellness is perhaps the most important factor in the quality of our health and the quality of our lives. It allows us to feel good about ourselves, to enjoy others, and to avoid or quickly recover from emotional stress. Mental wellness also has a remarkable effect on how we prevent and recover from physical injury and illness.

Good mental health is being happy and liking yourself. You accomplish this by taking all the responsibility to make yourself happy. This responsibility includes your ability to adapt your thoughts, behaviors, and feelings to help you make yourself happy and to help you cope during emotional upsets. No one else "makes" you happy, you do it yourself.

When you develop mental wellness you experience more than just the absence of problems. You build a surplus of good feelings and positive attitudes so that stressful situations can be handled without adverse effects on your health. You face problems as they arise and move on with your life.

Mental wellness is fostered by a family life where every member is made to feel worthwhile and fulfilled. Members of the family need to encourage others to feel good about themselves. Parents must remember that they are as important as their children, and deserve the good feelings that come with mental wellness. Besides, fostering positive attitudes in others is easier when you feel good about yourself.

You are the one most likely to observe a problem in family members. Your support may be needed to help them return to mental wellness, just as you may from time to time need their support to work through problems of your own. However, no one can provide happiness for another person. You can simply help a person solve problems as they go through life seeking mental wellness.

The purpose of this chapter is to provide you with practical guides on how to recognize when your mental health or that of another needs some extra support. Mental health problems are no different than any others. Most are minor and caused, faced, and resolved in the process of everyday living. Others require a more conscious and concentrated effort and often a little help from friends or family. Relatively few require expert assistance or outside resources to resolve. It is hoped that this chapter will help you deal with all three stages—from increasing the wellness boosters you give and receive in daily life to deciding when you should seek the help of a counselor or mental health professional.

The early part of the chapter deals with recognizing symptoms of emotional problems and determining whether a problem is really a problem or simply a temporary indication that a person is coping with a stressful situation. Later, the chapter turns to basic prevention and self-care for mental health problems including practical advice on using open communication as a primary approach to helping someone work through an emotional problem. Finally, guidelines are provided on when to seek help from mental health professionals.

Symptoms of Emotional Problems

When a person experiences an emotional problem, it usually surfaces in the form of one or more common symptoms. The person appears anxious or depressed, hostile or withdrawn, or exhibits some other change in behavior. By learning to recognize these symptoms you increase your ability to help the person understand and resolve the basic problem.

Anyone, at any age, can experience emotional problems. In observing your family, don't dismiss symptoms in a toddler because you feel she is too young to have problems. The most common emotional symptoms are discussed below. Your understanding and recognition of them should help you in maintaining and restoring mental wellness in yourself and your family.

ANXIETY

Anxiety is an undefined fear. Fear is a normal, useful emotion which warns you when you are in danger. If you are driving and are almost struck by another car, you experience fear. This fright helps you react and you swerve to miss the other car. After a while you will return to your normal emotional and physical state.

Anxiety is the presence of fear but with the absence of an obvious or immediate source of danger, such as a near collision. Anxiety is characterized by all or any combination of the following symptoms: restlessness, shortness of breath, inability to concentrate, sleeplessness, a pounding heart, a feeling of weight on your chest, and general nervousness. It can also be revealed in physical complaints such as headaches, stomach cramps, muscle tension, or irritable bowels. Since you cannot see what is endangering you, you cannot do anything directly to deal with it, such as you did when you swerved to miss the other car. It is very difficult to return to your normal resting state without the symptoms of anxiety because you can't deal directly with your fears.

Anxiety can be approached from 2 directions. The most direct approach is to identify and resolve the undefined fear. When the anxiety has developed quickly or seems to be tied to a particular set of events this may be the best approach. Unfortunately, anxiety is more often caused by a complex set of sources which may relate to many different aspects of a person's life. In such cases improved relaxation may provide the best solution.

Anxiety often builds upon itself. If you feel anxious about a final exam or drivers' test you may think that there must be something for you to worry about. This new worry may cause your anxiety to increase even more. In such cases relaxation can do more than just treat the surface symptoms. Employing relaxation techniques as soon as anxiety is noticed can prevent the problem from getting out of hand. Such on-the-spot relaxation combined with regular relaxation or meditation practices can do much to make life easier and more enjoyable. Some relaxation exercises are described on page 204.

DAYDREAMING

Daydreaming from time to time and fantasizing about accomplishments is common. Such daydreaming is often a positive beneficial time out from stressful demands of everyday life. Some people, however, seem to live in their daydreams more than in real life. Daydreaming in school may be one response of a passive child who is having trouble with classwork, fears failure, and thus experiences anxiety. For that child daydreaming is an escape from anxiety. A child who daydreams only at home may be experiencing anxieties related to home life. Adults also daydream to escape frustration and anxieties. Daydreaming becomes a problem both with adults and children only when they spend more time in their dream world than in the real one.

HOSTILITY

Hostility is more than being temporarily angry at someone or something. It is a constant anger at the world in general, expressed through hostile actions. A hostile person may be physically or verbally aggressive against other people or things. This might include hurting other people by insulting, hitting, humiliating, scratching, embarrassing, or kicking them. Hostile people may also destroy property belonging to others or to themselves. Most hostile people learned this method of expression or anger from someone they used as a role model. If you pattern yourself after a hostile person, you will likely express anger in a hostile manner.

SELF-STIMULATION BEHAVIORS

Self-stimulation behaviors include head banging, hair sucking, nail biting, thumb sucking, and scratching. Of course, most children exhibit one or more of these behaviors at some time in their lives, but only for short periods of time. One cause of this type of behavior might be a lack of environmental stimulation. An example of this is a child's room with little color in it. You might try adding color to your child's room with pictures or posters. If the behavior is kept up for a long period of time, it may indicate there is anxiety in your child's life.

A child who has given up a self-stimulation behavior but returns to the behavior later deserves your attention. This can be a clue to you that your child is experiencing some type of stress. A child whose pet has died may return to a previous behavior, for example. This behavior alerts you to how your child is reacting to the loss.

When an adult exhibits a self-stimulation behavior, it may be the result of a habit which no longer stems from anxiety or an expression of anxiety.

DEPRESSION

There are basically two types of depression; reactionary and progressive. Reactionary depression occurs as a reaction to an event such as the death of a loved one. Other causes include the loss or sense of loss of a loved one, a job, self-esteem, or any other life situation that is viewed as a personal loss. Progressive depression is feelings of sadness or disappointment for no apparent reason. It can be caused by frustration, unexpressed anger, or by an inability to live up to expectations of yourself or of others. Both types of depression must be dealt with; time doesn't necessarily heal all wounds unless accompanied by some action.

Common symptoms of depression include fatigue, a change in sleep habits, inability to concentrate, restlessness, boredom, lack of interest in food or sex, and feelings of helplessness, apathy, hopelessness, despair, and discouragement. The depressed person usually cannot recognize what to do about the depression.

It is sometimes difficult to see depression in children. They may mask the symptoms by with- drawing, as described on page 186.

Depression ranges from feeling "blue" to having all the above symptoms. Feeling "blue" is nor- mal in such cases as failing an exam or being criticized by your employer. More severe depression needs your special understanding and home care, especially if you have noticed any of the above symptoms for a while. Prolonged depression is a serious problem that may require professional help, since continual feelings of worth- lessness can lead to impaired func- tioning and an inability to get along with other people. It is important that the depressed person's lost feel- ings of personal value and worth are restored.

For some cases of mild depres- sion you may be able to help by giving psychological wellness boosters as discussed on page 187. Also the mildly depressed person may be able to revive feelings of personal value and worth by in- teraction with new people. Help ar- range introductions to other people and encourage the person to meet new people.

HYPERACTIVITY OR EXCITEMENT

Each of us becomes excited about some events in our lives. It is normal to feel excited about birth- days, holidays, or other special events. Hyperactivity, meaning "more activity than normal," refers to continuous symptoms such as the inability to sit still in one place or the jumbling of ideas and thoughts to the point that a per- son's speech is not clear. Because "normal" activity levels change as a child grows older, hyperactive symptoms should be measured against what is normal for other children of the same age.

The causes of hyperactivity are varied. In rare cases these symp- toms are directly related to an un- derlying physical disorder and may be accompanied by other signs of illness, such as dramatic mood changes, lack of coordination, learning disorders, and short atten- tion span. Those with a physically based hyperactivity can usually benefit from medical evaluation and care.

Diet and drugs are thought to play a role in some cases where there are hyperactive symptoms. Research suggests that antihis- tamines and food additives can cause or increase hyperactivity in some people. Reduction in the con- sumption of sugar or caffeine can sometimes be effective in alleviating hyperactive symptoms.

More often the cause of hyperac- tivity is either unknown or psycho- logical in nature. Frequently, it is directly related to anxiety or frus- tration. Mental stress should be suspected, particularly when the symptoms occur at school or work but not at home, or at home but not at school. Also suspect a stress reaction if someone is able to sit through a favorite television program, but not able to sit still at other times.

WITHDRAWAL

Most of us at times need to get away from the crowd and be alone. Some people, however, continually seek to avoid other people. Typically, people who withdraw talk less than they used to, stay in their rooms or homes more, play with other people less, or participate less in a group they formerly enjoyed. Frequently missed practices or games with a child's baseball team may be an example of withdrawal. These people literally withdraw from society. There are three basic reasons for withdrawal. The first, depression, is the most common reason for withdrawal. The second is the feeling "no one wants to be with me," so they withdraw from everyone. Thirdly, anger may cause withdrawal. When passive or shy people experience constant anger, they may deal with that anger by withdrawing.

When a Problem Is a Problem

Sometimes a person will exhibit an emotional problem that is temporary. This doesn't always indicate a problem which needs attention. All of us may exhibit temporary fears and anxiety as we seek to perform well at new activities. How do you know when symptoms are serious? There are four rules of thumb that you can go by which apply to adults and to children.

- If any symptom becomes a *continued or permanent pattern of a person's behavior,* you should become concerned. If your daughter sucks her thumb or bites her nails in a stressful situation, she probably doesn't have a problem. If she always has a thumb in her mouth or always bites her nails, she may need some extra help. If a business associate who occasionally closes her door to be alone begins to keep it closed all day, you should be aware that her mental wellness may need a booster.

- When symptoms become *numerous,* be suspicious that there may be a problem. For example, if your son entering school exhibits several concurrent symptoms such as fighting, refusing to go, and poor learning skills, he may need assistance. Any one of these symptoms alone would cause little concern unless it lasted an extended period.

- People need help if any symptom begins to *interfere with the ability to maintain normal behavior routines*. Examples of this are if they become antisocial or excessively withdrawn or aggressive. Symptoms of depression following the loss of a job are normal and need not be considered a mental health problem as long as the person is able to cope with family and friends. The person still, of course, needs your tender, loving care. However, signs of withdrawal from normal relationships in these areas should signal the need for special concern, assistance, and home care. Sleeping in occasionally is not a sign of being unable to handle daily activities. You should be concerned when a spouse or child remains in bed continually, for days, to escape the activities around them.

- Whenever an *existing pattern of behavior becomes excessive or extreme*, it should be considered a sign of an underlying problem. For example, a child who tends to be shy may reach the point of completely shunning friends and family. Another example is truancy from school or work. An occasional day missed isn't a problem, but many days can indicate a problem.

Prevention

Prevention of mental health problems is just as important as prevention of physical illness. The love and attention you give your family members is the best prevention. One way to monitor how much attention family members are receiving is by using psychological boosters. Think about the last few days. How many times did you tell your child or spouse, "Stop doing that," "No," "Because I said so"? How many times did you give psychological boosters such as "You did a good job of setting the table," "You look very nice today," or "Thank you"? Everyone needs some boosters and life is much more pleasant if the boosters outweigh the putdowns and negative comments. Try out some psychological boosters on yourself and your family.

Getting enough psychological boosters can raise your mental well "quotient." So, too, can limiting your exposure to life stresses. Stressful events, if they become more than you can adequately cope with, can lead to feelings of anxiety, mental health problems, and even physical illness.

It's easy to understand this. If your "mental wellness quotient" is high, you're apt to view a minor upset as minor and deal adequately with it. Even a major problem won't be a crisis to a woman who is feeling good about herself and her life. But when many major events in our lives happen all at once, the tension levels build and coping becomes more difficult.

Major events that may be viewed as stressful include both positive and negative experiences. The death of a spouse, divorce, or a major illness rank among the most stressful. Marriage and the birth of a child also rate high. If you have recently experienced such an event or many lesser changes such as moving, starting a new job, or starting school, you should realize that you are at a much higher risk of health problems. It isn't realistic to think you can avoid these major events, although you might be able to postpone some. However, recognizing that you have undergone many changes and cannot avoid some more, you can prepare yourself. Clear your calendar. Plan for more free time. Increase your outlets for relieving tension and improve your relaxation and coping skills. See page 204 for planned relaxation exercises and treat yourself to relief from muscular tension. You might also try communication with someone to talk about the changes you are experiencing and how you feel about the changes.

THE 4 SQUARES*

One good method of looking at your life and those of your family members to observe stressful changes, is by employing the 4

* Developed by John E. O'Malley, M.D., Harvard Medical School

Squares. The 4 Squares represent 4 major areas of a person's life. The structure of the 4 Squares can give you an approach to looking at a person's life, as a monitoring tool during the regular home physical exam or to help discover a suspected problem. The Squares can help you discover how things are going in each area of a person's life—about the same, getting better, or deteriorating. If anything is upsetting mental wellness or any area of a person's life needs psychological boosters, it is likely to show up in one of these squares.

Square 1: Work or School: Notice if the person is always being late for or missing appointments, constantly complaining about their jobs or class, dragging their feet every morning about getting ready, not achieving a measure of success that is at their level of growth, or having unusual difficulties concentrating even when there are no distractions.

Square 2: Family: Observe if the person is bossy and trying to control the lives of others in the family or if they are always being picked on by other family members or being put down in some way. Does the person feel accepted and liked by the family?

Square 3: Friends or Acquaintances: Healthy people have friends they can trust. Observe if the person treats friends as if they are enemies by always being suspicious of friends' motives or by not trusting them.

Square 4: Self: Observe how people refer to themselves. Is it always a cutting remark? Can they never seem to receive a compliment? Do they make derogatory remarks about themselves?

The Squares work best with open communication. They help you *focus* on an area of a person's life, but only communication can determine whether or not a problem exists. Whether you observe a problem and ask a question about it—"Are you unhappy at school?" or ask a leading question—"How are things going with the boss?", or make a statement a person must refute or confirm—"You seem to have a really good friend in Jim," depends on the lines of communication you have opened.

Home Care

Understanding, acceptance, empathy, and communication are generally your best methods of home care. To be understanding you need to be aware of the person's personality, environment, and have a knowledge of causes and symptoms of stress. Two people can face the same situation differently; one person is able to cope, the other person only sees and feels stress. If you understand the person you are dealing with, you can better relate her or his particular personality or environment to the current mental health difficulties.

Acceptance means looking beyond the image that the troubled person presents and seeing the total

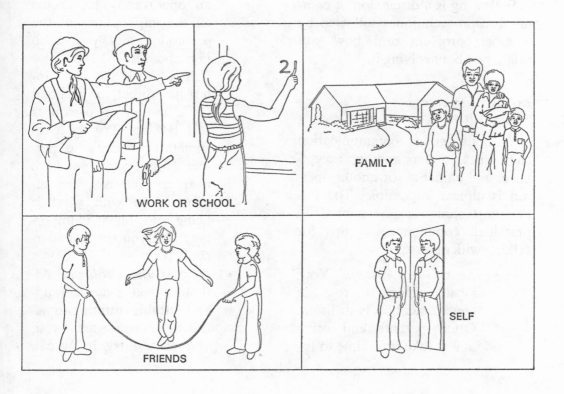

worth of the person as a human being. This can be especially difficult if the problem is socially unacceptable, eg., alcoholism or promiscuous behavior.

Empathy is realizing that although the person may not exhibit any physical signs of an illness, he or she nevertheless is experiencing true pain. If you are feeling mentally well, it may be easy for you to impatiently say "Cheer up" or "Snap out of it" to a troubled person. This doesn't help the person and, in fact, may make her or him feel more troubled and even guilty.

Good communication is essential to any relationship and is certainly very important during troubled times. Development of good communication techniques is invaluable in your dealings with others.

Following is a discussion of communication techniques followed by a mock problem and how you might go about solving it.

COMMUNICATION TECHNIQUES

Without good communication techniques, understanding, acceptance, and empathy for another person is almost impossible. The following techniques are offered as practical, common sense tips for talking with others.

- *Learn to Listen:* Your most important role in communication is to listen. Often parents and other adults take little time to lis-

ten because they are too busy lecturing, giving advice, or talking about their own similar experiences. If you learn the technique of listening, you may be better able to draw out the person talking. The person may be more apt to relate feelings to you rather than events. Your part in listening is to maintain eye contact and an interest in what is being said. If your spouse tells you she or he is in line for a big promotion at work, your first reaction should be "How do you feel about that?" rather than asking details of the promotion itself. Later, of course, will come an opportunity to discuss all the implications of the promotion and your feelings about it.

It is best if you don't interrupt, direct, or respond while the other person is still talking. Try to learn something about the person from what you are hearing. You may not always agree with what is being said, but it is important that you try to understand it.

- *Restate the Problem:* Although you may feel uncomfortable restating something someone tells you, you should try it. It can sometimes amaze you that you aren't talking about the same problem. If your son tells you he's been having trouble fighting the kids in school, be sure he's not talking about a good natured wrestling match before you get too concerned about his mental health.

- *Lecture Less:* If you lecture to someone, she or he is likely to become defensive. If your child is fighting with other children, ask, "Why are you fighting?", rather than saying, "Don't fight." A question asked in this manner may have two benefits. First, the child may stop fighting and second, your child may open an avenue of communication by telling you why she or he is fighting.

- *Putting Yourself in the Other Person's Shoes:* Think in terms of the person having the problem. Try to remove yourself from your own feelings and think of the other person. Ask yourself some questions, such as: "Why does the person seek to solve problems in this particular way?" "Are they afraid of someone?", "Are they daydreaming because they are afraid of failing

and don't want to try?", "Why are they so angry?"

- *Consider Your Role in the Problem:* Ask yourself what part you play in the other person's problems. Am I being too strict or too restrictive? Am I too demanding? Have I communicated messages that say I don't care and am indifferent?

- *Try to Meet Anger with Calmness:* One of the biggest traps facing family communication is the blow-up syndrome. If your teenager is expressing anger at you, try to understand it. Restrain your impulse to strike back. When you respond with anger, the chances for further communication and solutions are diminished. Also, your calmness may help calm down the other person.

- *Be Sure It's Not Your Problem:* An important part of communication is to realize that sometimes you, as the parent, own the problem. One example of this is your negative reaction to a teenager choosing to go to a trade school rather than college. If you feel reluctant because you want all your children to be college graduates, then you own the problem. Similarly, don't fret about your daughter's mental health because she starts dreading piano lessons. If you are the force behind the lessons consider the possibility that the problem may be yours.

- *Use a Go-Between:* Sometimes it may be difficult for you to get your child to communicate with you, especially if you haven't communicated in a long time. If your child is being uncooperative, try waiting a while and try not to keep pushing. If you still can't start communications try getting a neutral person to intervene. This person may be a teacher, counselor, clergy member, sibling, or a family friend that your child respects. Another method you might try is to suggest that your children write down their feelings. They can then organize their thoughts and not be interrupted by you. Children can also symbolize their feelings by drawing how they feel.
- *Accept the Person's Feelings:* When your children relate their feelings to you, don't make judgments. Feelings are neither bad nor good and everyone should have a right to experience them. If your daughter claims she hates her

baby brother, this may be a valid expression of her present attitude. Don't say, "Of course you don't hate him" and make her feel guilty for her feelings. A better approach would be to say, "How do you feel toward him right now?" or "I understand how you might feel that way sometimes." Let her express her anger, jealousy, or whatever it is she is feeling.

- *Know When You Need Help:* When you are helping anyone, keep your own limitations in mind. Emotional problems are not easy to deal with, especially when they are related to your own relationships. Sometimes the help of parents, spouse, or friends isn't enough. This can be especially true if the problem has remained unsolved for too long. When this happens, it is time to call for expert help from a mental health professional.

HELPING SOLVE A PROBLEM

Keeping communication techniques in mind, here is an example of how to help solve a mental health problem. Your son Jeff seems depressed to you: he appears restless, bored, sad, and discouraged. The first thing to do is try to find out the reason for his depression. Sometimes this takes a lot of effort. Talk to Jeff, utilizing the communications techniques above. The 4 Squares concept may help you narrow the problem to one particular area of his life. If, after several attempts, your son still won't tell you, you may need to talk to his teachers, school counselor, his friends, or others to help find the problem. After finding out that Jeff is depressed because he has lost self-esteem through flunking a course in school, you need to help Jeff realize that his depression is related to the flunking problem. Lots of people with depression and anxiety cannot determine the cause by themselves and need the help of a neutral person to point it out to them.

After relating the cause to the depression, it's time to start solving the problem with your child. Ask Jeff how he thinks the flunking problem could be solved. You and he might decide he needs to readjust his study habits, have you help more with his homework, and both of you meet with his teacher to seek more solutions such as retaking tests.

It may work out that Jeff does or does not flunk the course. The important point is that as a parent you gave support and understanding to your son. His mental health can only benefit from your consideration.

When to Call a Health Professional

If you feel your interactions aren't working, it's time to obtain help from a mental health professional. You may be doing everything possible for your child or yourself and doing it well, but maybe you just didn't zero in on all of the problem. Sometimes all you need is another opinion to help you back on the right track. Of course, after seeking help, your understanding, acceptance, and support is just as important as it was before you sought help.

Another reason to seek professional help is if your own problems are interfering with your helping your child. If you are suffering from depression, you may be less likely to notice withdrawal in your child. You may be even less likely to be able to help. If you can see problem symptoms in yourself, you should realize that they make you less able to help your child, and may need professional help for both you and your child.

Notice if there are classes on communication, stress reduction, or relaxation being offered in your area. These could be an effective alternative to counseling.

A mental health professional can be anyone who can expertly listen to you. The person can either help you solve problems or refer you to someone who can. Don't be discouraged and stop seeking help just because the person you talked with the first time wasn't helpful. Help for you to help yourself is available somewhere. Don't try to find someone to solve your problems for you. Only you can do that. But a qualified person can help *you* solve your own problem.

Places to seek help are the local mental health center, mental health association, your clergy, or a school guidance counselor. Depending on your needs, you may be referred to a psychiatrist, psychologist, social worker, or other qualified counselor.

Don't stop yourself from seeking help because of what other people might think. You should feel free to use whatever resource you think would be helpful in the resolution of your emotional concerns.

Promoting Mental Wellness

Life is filled with stressful situations and at some time or another, either you or someone you care about will have difficulty in coping. Hopefully, this chapter will help you during troubled times. Remember, though, that good mental health is much more than the absence of problems. Seek good mental health for yourself. A mentally healthy person has a good self image, expresses feelings, can cope with bad news, and enjoys life to its fullest. Life feels good to a mentally healthy person.

12

Becoming Healthwise

For most of us, our health becomes apparent only when we lose it: when a bad cold makes us feel miserable or a backache puts us in bed for a few days. The preceding chapters of this handbook have presented guidelines for recognizing and responding to these minor health problems that interrupt our day-to-day routines. By following these guidelines, a parent can confidently deal with family health problems in an effective and rewarding way.

But being "healthwise" is much more than just responding to problems as they arise. To be healthwise is to recognize that in the long run our health is most affected by the way we choose to live. This chapter will help you review your own living routine and examine its positive and negative effects on your health. Unlike the first chapters, there are no guidelines to follow and no suggestions of when to see a health professional. Your life is your own

and you alone must decide how important good health is to you.

Once we choose to, there are many ways to reduce the risks of poor health. By not smoking, by eating wisely, and by following basic safety rules we can strengthen our chances for a long and healthy life. The discussion in this chapter is centered on exercise and stress, 2 risk factors with significant effects on our health. These factors are highlighted because they are so closely linked to how good we feel and how much we enjoy our lives. For many people the way they cope with stress and the time they devote to useful exercise may become the most important keys for a healthier life.

In the last section of the chapter you will be invited to write a prescription for your health. It must take into account the goals, values, and barriers of your own life. It is a prescription that no doctor or other professional can write for you.

Hopefully, that prescription will become your personal plan for a longer, healthier life.

Exercise

Exercise is the way we use our bodies. If muscles and organs aren't used or exercised, they lose their capacity to work. To stay healthy we all need to exercise to some degree. This section will help you review the ways you put your own body to work and the benefits you expect or would like to get in return. Your own analysis of how you exercise and why will lead to a major component of your prescription for health.

Most people kid themselves about how much exercise they really get. The farmer who used to stay in top shape from endless chores and hard work may not realize that a gradual change from manual labor to machinery has lightened routine exercise patterns. Similarly, an active wife may gradually give up her own exercise patterns for the growing needs of her young family.

WHY PEOPLE EXERCISE

Many people get exercise because they can't avoid it. Their job may require hard physical work or they just get exercise as an unnoticed part of their daily routine. Historically, this routine exercise has served to keep most people "in shape."

Others get exercise as part of their recreation and entertainment. Sports, hikes, or dancing are usually done just for the fun of it and without much thought of the physical benefits. Unfortunately, however, many people find exercise becoming a smaller and smaller part of their lives. Spectator sports either in person or on TV have cut deeply into more active recreational patterns. Labor-saving devices have saved us from exercise both on the job and at home.

More today than at any other time, exercise has become a decision. We must consciously choose activities that support our physical need for conditioning if we wish to reap the benefits that conditioning can bring. People must recognize and value these benefits before their exercise patterns can be strengthened.

Perhaps the single most important reason people choose physical activity is that it makes them feel good. Exercise in reasonable regular amounts invigorates the body and relaxes the mind. It also makes you look good. The muscle tone and fitness of a conditioned person at any age is always admired.

Some people exercise to help them relax from tension or to assure restful sleep. Rest is the body's natural reaction to exercise and is part of the conditioning process.

Others perceive exercise as a way to control their weight. The more calories that are used in exercise, the more you can eat without gaining weight.

Increasingly, people are choosing to become more conditioned expressly to strengthen their hearts. Their exercise patterns aim at improving the heart muscle and the blood flow to the heart.

BARRIERS TO EXERCISE

Whatever the reasons for your own physical activities, there are always barriers that work to limit the amount of exercise you get. Today time is the biggest barrier to regular exercise. We ride in cars and elevators rather than walk to save time. We can't take time for morning exercises. We can't get away for a regular tennis game or a hike with the family.

A second barrier to exercise is the feeling that we're just too tired. At the end of a tense day we just want to plop down and relax, usually in front of the television. We're much too tired to go for a swim or to play ball even though such activity would probably help relax us and restore our energy.

Embarrassment is a significant barrier to many people. Those not in good condition are often afraid that others will make fun of them. They're embarrassed at their appearances, their abilities, or both.

Another significant barrier to many people is the lack of someone to exercise with. This is critical in competitive sports and is a real disadvantage in developing a regular exercise pattern around team activities.

Weather is also a barrier, particularly for the person who is limited to a specific sport or outdoor activity. Regular skiing or ice skating in the winter must be combined with summer sports to assure a year-round program.

Many exercise activities are costly. Sports equipment, club memberships, or getting into a skating rink may be too expensive to handle on a regular basis. If less costly activities are not substituted for such expensive ones, the regular conditioning program will suffer.

YOUR EXERCISE PROFILE

An analysis of how and why you exercise will be useful to you later in this chapter. The following table is designed to help you construct your own exercise profile. First read the list of sample activities on the left. Mark each activity which you do often. Add any activities you wish.

Next estimate how much time you actively spent in each marked activity in the past 2 weeks. Mark the amount in minutes in column A.

In column B note any special benefits which help motivate you to participate in the activities. A list of possible benefits is presented at the bottom of the table.

Finally, note in column C any barriers which commonly prevent or limit your ability or desire to participate in the marked activities. Again, a list of possible barriers is provided.

Personal Exercise Profile

Check any of the following way/ways in which you often get exercise	A Estimate how much time you spent at activity during past 2 weeks	B List any benefits you would expect to get	C List barriers which keep you from doing activity
ROUTINE EXERCISE • Walk to work, store, etc. • Walk upstairs • Job requires exercise • Lawn care/gardening • Scrubbing/housework • Others (name)			
RECREATIONAL EXERCISE • Team sports such as basketball, volleyball, etc. • Individual competitive sports such as tennis, hand-ball, etc. • Non-competitive sports such as hiking, skiing, biking, etc. • Dancing • Others (name)			
FITNESS PROGRAM • Jogging, running, jumping rope, etc. • Calisthenics • Special exercises • Others (name)			

DESIRED BENEFITS FROM EXERCISE

1. Makes you feel good, look good.
2. Helps you sleep, relax.
3. Feeling of accomplishment.
4. Want to strengthen heart.
5. Helps you lose weight (calorie balance) Others (name).

SOME BARRIERS TO EXERCISE

1. Not enough time.
2. Too tired.
3. Embarrassed.
4. No one to do it with.
6. Bad weather.
6. Costs too much.
7. Never learned to enjoy exercise. Others (name).

Review your exercise profile thoughtfully. Later you may wish to consider it in planning how you might improve your health.

How much exercise a person should get depends on how great he or she needs each of the benefits listed in the Personal Exercise Profile. If you like to eat a lot, but wish to maintain a certain weight, you will need to burn the extra calories with exercise. For example, a brisk 1½ mile walk will burn about 100 calories, about the same amount in 1 slice of buttered toast.

Heart and circulatory improvements are other major reasons for exercising. Regular physical activity is known to strengthen the heart muscle, and open more blood vessels in the heart and other parts of the body. All this may mean decreased chance of heart disease. But how much exercise is needed to receive these benefits?

Since you are really exercising your heart, you should pay close attention to your pulse rate during exercise. The chart on page 200 presents a target pulse range during exercise for various age groups. It is believed that exercise must place your pulse into this range in order to effectively improve your circulatory system. Exercise at lesser rates is certainly good for you but will do comparatively less for your circulatory system. Sustained exercise over the target limits may fatigue and even damage the heart muscle.

For maximum impact on the circulatory system, an exercise session should start with a 5 minute warm-up to prevent injuries and soreness before reaching the target pulse range. Usually 20 minutes in the target range will then provide a significant conditioning effect on the cardiovascular system. Each session should also end with a 5 minute cool-down period in which the intensity of exercise is gradually reduced. This will usually prevent dizziness or nausea.

Ideally, a 30 minute exercise session such as has been described should be done 3 or more days per week.

EXERCISE CAUTION

An exercise program should begin gradually, especially for a person accustomed to limited physical activity. Start with exercise sessions below the target pulse range and of less duration. Then gradually increase the intensity and length of each session until you are able to safely stay within the target range for the prescribed 20 minutes.

Jumping into a rigorous exercise program without gradual conditioning is asking for trouble. Ten percent of males over age 35 have hidden heart disease that could be triggered by the sudden shock of vigorous exercise.

You should stop exercising and call a physician if any of the following symptoms occur:

- a sudden burst of rapid heartbeats.

Maximal Attainable Heart Rate and Target Zone
[Averages Only]

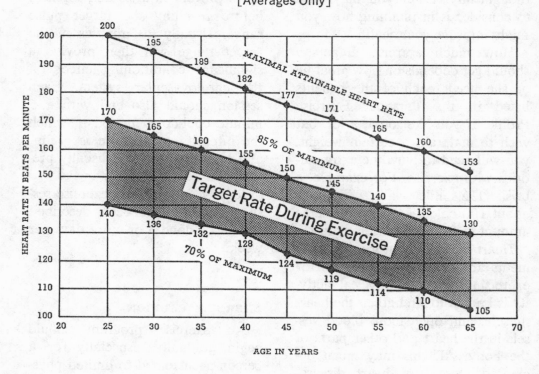

AGE IN YEARS

- a very slow pulse when a moment before it had been in the target range.
- pain or pressure in the center of the chest or the arm or throat related to exercise.

Coping and Relaxation

Stress is an emotional and physical condition that occurs whenever our feelings of security are disturbed. The body's normal stress response is to stimulate the heart rate, increase respiration, tense the muscles, and increase physical strength.

When physical danger induces stress, the body's stress reaction may be needed to divert the crisis. Then, when the danger has passed, the body relaxes and returns to its normal routine. Nearly everyone has felt that primitive fright when confronted by a vicious dog or shaken by an automobile collision.

In today's society, however, most dangers are more complex. Financial insecurity and emotional uncertainties are the threats to survival. Although the threats are no longer physical, the body still reacts in a physical way. Muscles tense and blood pressure rises as the body prepares for the danger, but the fight rarely comes. This continuous physical reaction without any real physical outlet is harmful to the body. It causes ulcers, headaches, and backaches and contributes to many other serious conditions such as heart disease. Stress may also reduce our resistance to colds and the flu. The degree of its impact on our health depends on how successful we are at recognizing and coping with stress.

RECOGNIZING STRESS

It's sometimes difficult to recognize or admit that stress is at work on your health. If you can learn to watch for the effects and to take corrective action quickly, you will be very much ahead in coping with your stress.

The signs of stress are classic. You get headaches, a stiff neck, or nagging backaches. You become irritable and intolerant of even minor disturbances. You lose your temper more and find yourself yelling at your children without real cause. Your pulse rate increases and you feel jumpy or exhausted all the time.

When such symptoms appear in you or in someone else, recognize them as signs of stress and think of a way to combat it. Just knowing why you're crabby may be the first step in coping with the problem. It is your attitude toward stress, not the stress itself, that most affects your health.

HOW TO AVOID STRESS

The best way to reduce stress is to eliminate or diminish its cause. This can be done either by removing yourself from the stressful environment or by controlling the environment to eliminate stress. People can think their way out of many stressful situations if they would only direct their attention to it. Most people never give themselves a chance.

To start the process, write on a piece of paper 2 regular situations that cause you stress. It may be a person who really upsets you, rush hour traffic, or the supermarket line when you're in a hurry. Income tax forms, bill paying, or a too-tight time schedule are also stressful to many people. Next, think about and answer the following questions about your problem:

- How can I avoid the situation?
- What can I do in advance to make the situation less stressful?
- Is it worth getting upset about or is it something I can take with a grain of salt or shrug off?

Don't be discouraged if your answers aren't helpful. Stress is sometimes very difficult to avoid. But sometimes the solution is easier than you imagine. Suppose for example that visiting a certain relative always upsets you because you get in disagreements about politics or the way you raise your children, or some other subject which you just don't want to discuss with that person. Since you probably don't want to avoid the relative altogether (or can't) think of ways to avoid the problem conversation areas. Make a list of topics you would like to talk to this person about and then be alert. Every time the talk drifts toward a stressful area, introduce a new topic to steer it away again. You may feel so happy with your success that the usual stress just won't develop. Even if the problem areas do arise, your more positive attitude may keep the stress from getting to you.

Stress avoidance can, of course, be overdone. Some people become so burdened by their stressful lives that they choose to just stay in bed all day and ignore it all. Clearly such people must develop new ways to cope with their problems.

HOW TO COPE WITH STRESS

For those problems that can't be avoided each one of us develops our own method of coping. If we are successful the stress and tension from a certain problem are short-lived and have little effect on our health. If we don't succeed in relieving stress, we may get headaches, digestive problems, high blood pressure, muscle aches, and other symptoms of physical illness.

Aside from avoidance there are 3 basic ways that people cope with stress: exercise, relaxation, and ex-

pression. Virtually everyone calls on all 3 forms to battle stress of one kind or another.

Exercise is a natural response to stress, the normal reaction to the fight or flight emotion. By running, for example, one can take advantage of the rapid pulse and tensed muscles caused by stress. The bundled up energy is expended in the exercise. After a long run, the stress emotions are much more easily relieved and returned to normal.

Relaxation is another natural method for coping with stress. To be effective, relaxation should allow you to rest your body and mind from stress. Ironically, relaxing isn't always as easy as it sounds. Most people consider a "relaxing" evening of television to be a good way to wind down after a stressful day. Unfortunately, watching a tense football game or suspense movie can sometimes keep the stress emotions on a slow boil all evening. For some people, reading a mystery thriller can also be stressful. Even sleep is not always relaxing, as anyone who has tossed and turned can attest. What is relaxing for one person may not be for the next.

Real relaxation can be found in a great variety of activities. Each person must find the methods which work best for that individual. Many people find the repetitive rhythms of knitting or fishing relaxing or the wholesome work of gardening a needed change of pace from the daily routine. For others, special relaxation techniques like yoga or meditation can release their tensions quickly before physical damage is done.

To be truly relaxing, an activity must allow the mind to slow down and release the things that cause stress. Unfortunately, many people have never stopped to develop good relaxation habits. Relaxing is a skill, but not a hard one to learn. Another short exercise may help.

Write down on a sheet of paper 2 ways that you are able to relax. Next ask the following questions about each method and make note of the answer:

- Does the method really refresh and relax you?
- Does it clear your mind and help you see things better?
- How long does it take to relax you?
- How often do you regularly get to relax in this way?

This brief exercise will help focus your attention on the important area of relaxation. If you could benefit from better relaxation habits, you need only prescribe them for yourself. Remember that the frequency and quality of relaxation is much more important than the duration or overall quantity. Since many people need a specific technique to help them relax, one is suggested on page 204.

A third way to cope with stress is through expression of feelings. Stress and tension affect our emotions and feelings. By expressing those feelings to others, we are able to better understand and cope with them ourselves. Crying can also serve to release tensions. It's part of our emotional healing process. Those people who develop a source of understanding in their spouse or good friend have an invaluable assistant in coping with stress in their lives. Expression through writing, crafts, or art may also be a good release.

CHEMICAL STRESS REDUCERS

In addition to our natural methods for reducing stress, many of us get additional assistance from chemical agents that help reduce or more often suppress stress. Whether these aids are as mild as aspirin for a tension headache or as powerful as narcotic drugs, their use points out weakness in our coping skills.

Coffee, cigarettes, alcohol, and both legal and illegal drugs are all part of the arsenal used against stress. Unfortunately, many of these substances have strong negative effects on the body. While they may temporarily relieve the symptoms of stress, they rarely resolve its underlying causes. Even more importantly, the use of these stress suppressants may block the development of positive coping skills and habits.

Simple Relaxation Technique

Of the many methods of relaxation and meditation the following 2 are among the simplest and most effective. Either should be done for about 15 minutes once a day (twice if you can). Pick a time and place where you won't be disturbed or distracted. You may wish to try one of the techniques for several weeks and chart your pulse rate before and after each session. Once you "get into" the relaxation process your pulse should decrease.

PROGRESSIVE RELAXATION TECHNIQUE—SUMMARY

Lie down on your back with your legs straight and your arms at your side. Use a small pillow for your head or a chair to rest your legs on if that's more comfortable. Close your eyes and take several deep breaths. Breathe with your abdomen as much as possible. Your stomach should rise and fall —not your chest. Place a hand on your stomach briefly to feel it move up and down.

Now you are ready to relax every part of your body. Start with your feet. Mentally tell them to relax. As you exhale each breath imagine that the air is flowing through your legs into your feet and relaxing them. You may experience a tingling or other sensations as you learn to relax.

Next, concentrate on your ankles and calves and repeat the mental

process. The purpose is to concentrate attention on one body part at a time until you can feel it relax. You should work progressively from the toes up through the thighs, buttocks, and lower back and then from the hands to the shoulders and lower back before going to the neck, face, and head. Continue to be aware of your abdominal breathing and to imagine the flow of exhaled breath going to warm and relax each part of you as you go through the exercise.

As you progressively relax your muscles, try to relax your mind. Be passive to thoughts as they come and go and try not to dwell on or think about any subject.

RELAXATION RESPONSE— SUMMARY

(For a fuller description see Herbert Benson's *The Relaxation Response*, 1975, Avon Books)

The second basic type of relaxation technique is one in which you repeat a chant, phrase, or sound which helps to block tension-producing thoughts which might otherwise come into your mind when you are relaxing. Transcendental Meditation (TM) is a widely known and used relaxation technique of this type. Although TM and other methods differ in exactly what is done they all are related to the general procedure discussed in the seven steps below.

1. Sit quietly in a comfortable position.
2. Close your eyes.
3. Deeply relax your muscles as described on page 204 under Progressive Relaxation.
4. Breathe from the abdomen and through the nose, remaining aware of your breathing. Breathe easily and naturally.
5. As you breathe out say the word "one" or "om" (rhymes with home) silently to yourself and repeat this for 10 to 20 minutes. As you passively repeat the word or sound, other thoughts will come into your mind. Try to neither dwell on nor shut out these thoughts. Just let them come in and out and return to the repetition of the sound.
6. When you finish sit quietly for a few moments with your eyes closed and later with your eyes open.
7. Practice the technique once or twice a day, but wait several hours after any large meal since digestion sometimes interferes with the relaxation response.

The regular practice of these techniques will begin to train your body in the art of relaxation. Developing this art can add a new and rewarding dimension to your life.

As you begin to feel tension in a stressful situation you will be able to call upon your art to maintain or restore a relaxed state of both body and mind. Learning to relax is one of the best ways to enjoy life more; it is an important part of becoming healthwise.

Your Diet and Your Health

In addition to the way we exercise and cope with stress, the way we eat has a great influence on our health. See the chapter "Eating Wisely" for ways to improve your nutrition. You may wish to include better eating habits as part of your self-prescription for better health.

Your Prescription for Health

As this chapter has emphasized, each individual is uniquely qualified to evaluate his or her own methods of exercise, relaxation, and coping. No one else can dictate what you should do with your time, what you should eat or drink, or how you should cope with your problems.

The chart on page 207 can now be filled out as your own self-prescription for better health. It should summarize your findings from the exercises and discussions presented in this chapter.

There are 6 major areas outlined

on the prescription form. You need not prescribe something for each one. Consider your limitations carefully and don't prescribe more than you can reasonably accomplish. On the other hand don't be afraid to challenge yourself to break old habits.

EXERCISE

Review your personal exercise profile on page 207. If you are concerned that you need more exercise pick out 1 or 2 of the activities you've checked and prescribe them to yourself on a regular basis. Be sure to consider both the benefits and barriers when indicating how each activity can best be done and what steps you can take to assure that it will be accomplished.

AVOIDING STRESS

Review the discussion about avoiding stress and your written responses to the questions on page 201. If you think you would benefit from learning improved relaxation methods or simply by relaxing more often, prescribe a remedy for yourself. Perhaps your prescription would be to enroll in relaxation classes you may have heard about, or to read a book or two to help you get started. What's important is to recognize whether or not you could benefit from better relaxation.

EXPRESSION

This one is difficult. Try to judge how well your relationships with other people allow you to get understanding and support for your problems. Also, look at how well you are able to support the coping abilities of others. Prescribe for yourself a plan to improve your expressions of feelings through friendships or through writing or art. You may get some help from the communications techniques discussed in Chapter 11.

CHEMICALS

The use of chemicals to relieve stress is discussed on page 203. If you think you would benefit from substituting exercise or relaxation for chemical stress remedies, prescribe how you might start such a substitution. For example, if you suffer from headaches you may wish to prescribe some specific relaxation exercises instead of aspirin. If you smoke reevaluate whether you now have a better basis for quitting.

DIET

Prescribe for yourself ways that you can accomplish changes in your diet that *you want* to make. If you're unsure about what's really good for you, prescribe some books to read or classes to attend on good nutrition and diet.

Your Prescription for Health

To promote a longer, healthier and happier life, I hereby prescribe that I shall follow the personal self improvement suggestions recommended below. I certify that by following these recommendations I will obtain benefits of health and well-being far in excess of the cost and energy expended in their attainment.

Signed, _____
Your Signature

Prescription — Recommended Actions	How I'll Do It
1. Exercise:	
2. Avoiding Stress:	
3. Relaxation:	
4. Expression of Feelings:	
5. Reducing Reliance on Chemicals:	
6. Diet:	
Other:	

Conclusion

Your prescription for health may be looking like a very big pill to swallow. You may have only enough time and energy to follow 1 or 2 parts of it at first. But remember, everything in that prescription reflects actions which you believe will benefit you. Although each part alone will help, only when all factors of your prescription are adopted are you assuming the full responsibility for your health. Only then will you begin to understand the feeling of being HEALTHWISE.

13

Your Home Health Center

The concept of a home health center can be a real asset as you take responsibility for family health. We suggest you develop a "center" of health information, supplies, drugs, and records, located in a specific place convenient for your family. Information includes this handbook and any other reference books on health you have. Supplies are tools such as a thermometer, tweezers, and humidifier. Page 209 has a discussion of recommended supplies. Drugs, both prescription and over-the-counter, are described on page 214. Records consist of family medical records of this handbook and any other written information on your family's health.

There are at least 3 reasons for starting and maintaining an organized, centralized location for all health care materials:

1. When an emergency or illness arises, you want to know what to do and have the necessary supplies and drugs for treatment.

2. If an accurate inventory is kept of all drugs and supplies, costly duplication can be avoided and you can be sure all supplies are fresh and ready.

3. Anyone who cares for your family, such as a relative or a babysitter, can easily be shown where everything is in case of a medical emergency.

The question of whether *every* home health care material must be stored in the same place is inconsequential. The key concept is that items must be readily found, and all responsible family members must know where everything is kept. Keeping an up-to-date inventory is quite important. But since every family and each home is different, there is no one best location.

Survey your home to decide what is most suitable. Variables which influence location include contents of the center and space available in your home. Some families don't need as much room since they have fewer articles in their centers. Pick a spot that is handy but that won't be cluttered up with other goods. A closet or a dresser drawer dedicated solely to health needs are examples of locations. In some families it may not be practical to literally have all medical needs in one place. Maybe records are kept with other books and drugs are stored separate from other bulky supplies such as the humidifier. This is okay as long as the concept for a home health center is realized.

If you have small children or if any visit you, you should consider their safety. Either lock the entire center or find a lockable box, such as a lockable fishing tackle box, to hold your drugs. Potentially dangerous supplies such as tweezers and scissors should also be inaccessible to small children. Keep them locked with your drug supply.

Home Health Center Supplies

Supplies for the home health center include tools needed to help you treat your family's medical problems. Some supplies, such as a thermometer and tweezers, are a must for every center. Others, such as a blood pressure cuff, are optional. You know your family's needs best and can determine which supplies you need. Below is a comprehensive list of suggested supplies. Each major item is discussed in the remainder of this chapter.

BULB ASPIRATOR OR BULB SYRINGE

The difference between a bulb aspirator and a syringe is the tip. The aspirator has a shorter tip than the syringe. Since they can be used interchangeably, you need only purchase one. The syringe may be easier to use, but care must be taken because of the longer tip. Misused, it could damage an infant's membranes.

Aspirators or syringes are used to remove the mucus from an infant's nose. Babies can't be taught to blow their noses, but the mucus still must be removed. Compress the air from the bulb, place the tip into the infant's nostril, and gradually release bulb pressure and the mucus will flow into the tip. Rinse it out and repeat as often as necessary.

DENTAL MIRROR

A dental mirror can be useful but is not necessary to examine teeth and gums. Your dentist may be able to give you one or you can purchase one at some drugstores.

Home Health Center Supplies

Supplies	Quantity or Size
Bulb aspirator or bulb syringe	1 ounce
Dental Mirror	
Disclosing tablets	30 tablets
First Aid Supplies:	
Adhesive strips ("Band-aids")	70 assorted
Adhesive tape	1 in. x 10 yds.
Cotton balls	250
Elastic bandage	3 in. x 126 in.
Roller gauze bandage	2 in. x 5 yds.
Safety pins	
Scissors	Small
Sterile gauze pads	15 md., 10 lg.
Heating pad	
Humidifier or vaporizer	1 gallon
Nail clippers:	
Toe	
Finger	
Penlight	
Stethoscope	
Sphygomoanometer or blood pressure cuff	
Thermometer	
Throat culture kit	
Tweezers	

DISCLOSING TABLETS

Disclosing tablets are used to check how well you are brushing and flossing your teeth. They are small red tablets that you chew up and swish around in your mouth. Any plaque on your teeth will then turn red. These tablets can be used to effectively teach children how to brush properly.

EYE DROPPER

An eye dropper is inexpensive but can be handy. You'll need an eye dropper to insert saline nose drops, discussed on page 224. Sometimes it is soothing to use drops of cool water in red, tired eyes.

FIRST AID KIT SUPPLIES

There are many places you need a first aid kit—in your car, tractor, backpack, office, boat, trailer, or bicycle. It can be expensive to buy a first aid kit for each of these locations. If you buy the kit's supplies in bulk and assemble the kits yourself, you can save money and include only those articles that are needed in each kit.

HEATING PAD

A heating pad is usually more convenient than a hot water bottle although each performs the function of providing warmth to a particular area of the body.

HUMIDIFIER OR VAPORIZER

Humidifiers and vaporizers are devices which add moisture to the air. A humidifier increases the moisture with a cool mist while a vaporizer puts out hot steam. The two terms, however, are sometimes used interchangeably. A humidifier has several advantages: it can't burn you, it makes tinier particles of water which can go further into the respiratory system, it can't hurt the furniture, and the cool air is more comfortable and doesn't "wilt" you. However, a humidifier is noisier than a vaporizer, and you need to clean it with a disinfectant cleaner after each use and rinse it thoroughly. A vaporizer's biggest disadvantage is that the hot water can give a severe burn to anyone who overturns it or gets too close.

Whichever you choose, your family can benefit from a humidifier or vaporizer. They increase the humidity in the air and moistened air has less tendency to dry sensitive membranes. Humidity in the air can soothe a scratchy throat, help the dry, hacking cough, and make it easier for a person with a stuffy nose to breathe. In general, moisturizing the air of a home will help anyone feel more comfortable, especially in the winter when the home is closed and artificially heated.

PENLIGHT

A penlight has a small intense light which can be easily directed.

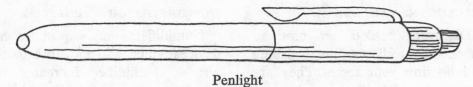

Penlight

It is useful while giving a physical exam and is easier to handle than a flashlight.

STETHOSCOPE

A stethoscope will make it easier for you to hear heart and chest sounds for a home physical exam. It is not an essential item for every home health center, however. If there is someone with hypertension in the family, then it's a good idea to have a stethoscope and a blood pressure cuff to frequently monitor their blood pressure. If you decide to buy a stethoscope, purchase the flat diaphragm model rather than the bell-shaped one. The flat diaphragm model makes it easier for you to hear.

SPHYGMOMANOMETER OR BLOOD PRESSURE CUFF

A sphygmomanometer is not an essential part of a home health center unless some member of the family is a diagnosed hypertensive. It is then needed to take frequent readings of blood pressure. A cuff can, of course, also be used to determine normal blood pressure and tell when the pressure is rising or abnormal. For a description of how to use a sphygmomanometer, see page 22.

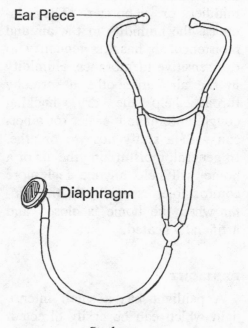

Ear Piece

Diaphragm

Stethoscope

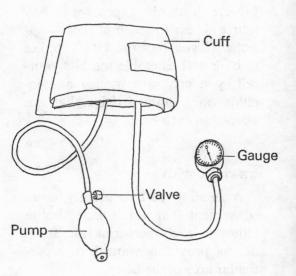

Cuff

Gauge

Valve

Pump

Blood pressure cuff

THERMOMETER

A thermometer is an important article in your home health center. If you have small children or for other reasons take rectal temperatures, it is suggested that you buy both an oral and a rectal thermometer. The rectal thermometer is fatter and thicker, so it breaks less easily. See page 19 for how to take a temperature.

THROAT CULTURE KITS

A throat culture kit consists of a swab, which looks like a large Q-tip, and a container which holds the swab. The kit is used when strep throat is suspected. If strep throats are a frequent occurrence in your family, or if you face the need of having your whole family cultured, you should investigate taking the throat swab yourself. You should be able to do an effective job once you are shown how it is done.

These kits are usually available at state health laboratories. Call your state lab to find out if they are available. You don't need to buy the swabs as their price is included in the culturing process by the lab. However, the labs ordinarily will not give you the results of the culture. You must still call your health professional for the results, but at least you will have saved the initial office visit to get a swab taken.

The kits may also be available at your health professional's office. They cannot be purchased at pharmacies.

TWEEZERS

Tweezers will be needed to remove foreign objects from the nose of a child. For symptoms of Object In Nose, see page 92. Buy the blunt-tipped type to avoid harming the membranes of the nose. You may also wish to buy regular sharp tweezers for removal of splinters.

14

Your Medicine Chest

Your medicine chest. What's in it for you?

KEEP TRACK OF YOUR DRUGS

First of all, take a look inside your medicine cabinet and anywhere else in the house you might keep drugs—the kitchen cupboard or windowsill, a purse, the nightstand. You'll probably find drugs the purpose of which you have long since forgotten, bottles, with labels half torn off, or with just a teaspoon or 2 of that cough syrup that helped Sue feel so much better last year—or was it 2 years ago? And, incidentally, did you find the aspirin? Or can't you recall exactly where you last put it?

The point is, *don't* hoard old drugs, and *do* keep those you need in a central location. It is also very important that you know what drugs you have on hand, what their purpose is, and how long they are effective (their shelf-life).

A form to help you keep an inventory of drugs on hand is in "Family Medical Records." Later in this chapter you will find information on how long certain drugs remain effective, and how best to store them.

For the most part, the drugs your family needs should be kept in a central location, so everything you need to maintain family health is easily accessible. These drugs, however, should be in a locked container if small children live in or visit your home. A medicine cabinet, "out of reach," is not out of reach to a curious, active child.

Exactly which drugs should you have on hand? There are as many answers to this question as there are health professionals. Actually, most of us need to keep few drugs on hand. The only real *must* is syrup of ipecac. This product is used to induce vomiting when someone has swallowed certain poisons. Aspirin is an old standby, yet in some cases it is overused. Even so, most people will want to keep aspirin available. But it is very important to keep it locked with other drugs. Other than these, the drugs you keep will depend on your family's health needs and perhaps the distance to a source of necessary drugs. Some other products which your family may wish to keep on hand are described on page 230.

All drugs should be kept in their original containers. The label should state what the drug is and its purpose. Be sure your pharmacist includes this information on all prescription labels.

HOW TO USE THE DRUG INVENTORY FORM

Each time you purchase a drug, whether by prescription or over-the-counter, record the drug name, date of purchase, etc., on the Drug Inventory Form on page 237 of "Family Medical Records." Keeping track of the drugs you use can help you quickly trace any possible ill effects from drug interactions and is a good way to make sure your drugs are not out-dated.

TYPES OF DRUGS

Any medication or preparation taken to relieve symptoms of illness or injury is a drug, not merely those products prescribed by a health professional. Drugs have different effects on different people. What may have worked great for a friend might cause an allergic reaction in you. This applies both to prescription (Rx) drugs and over-the-counter (O-T-C) drugs, but generally it is assumed that O-T-C drugs are less likely to have bad effects on people. They are usually less powerful drugs or in weaker doses. That is why they are available to be taken without the consent and supervision of a physician. Nevertheless, O-T-C products are drugs and their possible ill effects should be studied before using them. The precaution section under each drug described in this chapter should help you determine if a drug's benefits outweigh the risk of ill effects.

Most of the drugs described in this chapter are over-the-counter products which can be purchased in any drugstore without a prescription. Occasionally, when only a prescription drug fits a particular need, that drug is noted. You will need to discuss these with your physician.

There are dozens of over-the-counter products for literally every symptom. How to decide which is best for you can be trying. This chapter lists some effective products, usually including the chief active ingredients. The brand names are given only as guides because other products may be just as good. If the ingredients are the same, ask your pharmacist to suggest a suitable product or let cost be the deciding factor. If you wish to further explore the world of over-the-counter products, *Without Prescription* is a valuable book which lists ingredients of many O-T-C products and suggests which ingredients are most effective for various symptoms. Written by Erwin Di Cyan, Ph.D. and Lawrence Hessman, M.D., the book is available in paperback (Simon & Schuster, 1972) and is a fascinating tour through the maze of products in every drugstore. A more recent book with lots of practical advice is *The People's Pharmacy,* by Joe Graedon (St. Martin's Press, 1976).

WHY USE DRUGS

The drugs described in this chapter are generally useful in alleviating the symptoms described. However, you should remember that there is a reason for particular symptoms occurring. Your body is reacting to some problem and it isn't wise to use a drug to mask the symptoms without trying to discover the underlying cause.

Sometimes, however, you know the problem is minor and will go away with or without treatment and you simply wish to relieve a symptom temporarily. Then it's good to know which drugs may help.

ON THE SUCCESS OF DRUG THERAPY

As medical science advances we learn amazing things about the power of the human mind. Even though great strides have been made in conquering disease with many newly-developed medications, a great deal of the success of drug therapy depends on the patient's attitude toward the drug. If a person thinks a drug is good it has a much better chance of working. This explains why placebos (pluh-see-bos), harmless pills containing no curative powers, are often as effective as indicated medications, and why people tend to recover more quickly with a prescribed medication than with the very same medication purchased over-the-counter.

This knowledge should help you heal yourself and your family faster. While medicines help your body heal, your attitude and your willingness to rest and let your body's healers work play a big role in recovery. Have faith in the medications you take and take them in the manner prescribed. You can help your health professional by asking whether a drug is really necessary and what its purpose is.

If your headaches go away even before the aspirin has a chance to dissolve, why not try simply relaxing and letting your body heal on its own? A glass of water may be just as effective.

Once you (or you with your health professional) decide that a drug is necessary for your illness, you must follow through by taking the drug as instructed. Be sure to ask your health professional for any special instructions about taking the drug: does 4 times a day mean during the waking hours only, or does it mean 4 times in 24 hours? You should know whether medication should be taken with meals or on an empty stomach, and whether certain foods may lessen the drug's effectiveness. Both your physician and your pharmacist should volunteer this information, but if they don't, ask.

Generally, "take with meals" means directly before, with, or after a meal. The medicine should at least be taken with some food, even if only a snack.

"Take without food" means the drug should be taken on an empty stomach. Take those drugs with water (not milk or juice) 1 hour before you eat or 2 hours after.

If you miss some doses, don't try to catch up by taking it all at once. Call your health professional to find out what to do. Even better, ask your health professional what to do about missed doses *at the time* the drug is prescribed.

Be sure also that your physician knows what other drugs, both prescription and over-the-counter, you are taking. Other drugs may not only weaken the effect of a prescribed medication, they may interact with the drug and cause a serious reaction in your body.

Remember, too, that alcohol is a drug which can react with many medications. The effect of alcohol taken with barbiturates or tranquilizers is not equal simply to a combination of the 2 effects. They react together and are much more powerful and unpredictable than separately.

Ask your physician or pharmacist what the expected side effects of the medication are. You will be less alarmed if you experience drowsiness or slight nausea if you know it is an expected side effect. If you have an unexpected reaction, or one that you feel is particularly severe for you, consult your health professional right away.

CONTROLLING COSTS OF MEDICATIONS

The cost of your medications should also concern you.

The most obvious way to control the costs of medications is to be certain the medication is necessary. When a prescription is written, ask your physician what it is for and what effects it will have. You should ask also if there is an over-the-counter product which would work just as well.

Another possible means of controlling costs is by buying generically. A generic is the general, non-brand classification of a drug product, as "facial tissue" is the generic of Kleenex. They are generally less expensive than brand name products and most are comparable to brand name products. Some generics, however, are less reliable in quality. You should ask your physician if there is a less expensive but equally effective generic drug available. Your pharmacist can select a reliable product if your physician prescribes generically.

If a drug is to be used for a chronic condition, you may sometimes save money by asking for a larger amount. Of course, be sure you would use the product before its potency expired.

SAFETY TIPS ABOUT DRUGS

Once you have a drug there are a few more things to remember:

- Keep all medications in their original containers.
- Store medications properly. Most should be kept cool and dry. Some should be refrigerated. Know the difference. Any medicine in a dark bottle is sensitive to light. If the bottle has been out a long time near light, dispose of it.
- Do not take medications in front of children. They are great mimics.

- Do not tell children that medicine is "candy." For this reason, candy-flavored medicine can be dangerous.
- Do not leave vitamins (particularly children's vitamins) on the dining table.
- Read the label before taking a drug. Many pills look alike. Turn on the light at night.
- Replace the cap tightly. Child-proof caps aren't child-proof if they aren't capped.

Drugs

The following section explains the value, purpose, and possible dangers of many common drugs.

Essential Drugs
Syrup of Ipecac

Optional Drugs for Symptomatic Relief
Anti-diarrheal Preparations
Aspirin and Acetaminophen
Cold Medications
Laxatives

Miscellaneous Medications
Antibiotics
Vitamins
General Purpose, Useful Medications

Essential Drugs in Your Home Health Center

SYRUP OF IPECAC

Syrup of ipecac (ip-uh-kack) is an over-the-counter drug which will cause a person to vomit quickly when it is swallowed.

In most cases of swallowed poison the best treatment is to get the substance out of the victim's stomach as quickly as possible. Syrup of ipecac is excellent for this.

Sometimes, causing the patient to vomit can be harmful. *Do not use ipecac if the patient has swallowed any of the following:*

- Alkalis, such as dishwasher detergents or cleaning solutions. Instead use diluted vinegar and follow with water and milk to neutralize.
- Petroleum distillates such as furniture polish, Kerosene, gasoline, oil-based paints, etc. Give water to

dilute the poison without inducing vomiting.

WITH ALL POISONINGS CALL YOUR DOCTOR, EMERGENCY DEPARTMENT, OR POISON CONTROL CENTER IMMEDIATELY.

DOSAGE FOR IPECAC

1 year to 3 years—1 tablespoon. 3 years to 6 years—2 tablespoons. You must follow with at least 12 ounces of water. This is essential to ensure vomiting. Try to keep the patient walking around.

Repeat in 20 minutes if the person has not yet vomited. Repeat only once. When the poisoning victim vomits, have the person lie on his or her side with mouth lower than chest so the vomited material will not re-enter the airway and cause more trouble. If the person leans over a toilet, be sure the chest is lower than the stomach.

The vomiting caused by ipecac is *very* violent and it should not be used in the following situations:

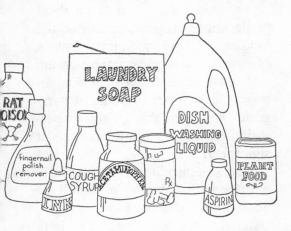

Induce vomiting

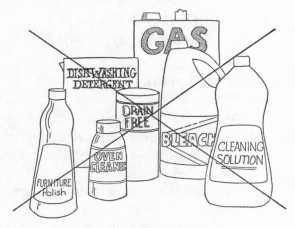

Do not induce vomiting

- If the victim is over 5 months pregnant.
- If the victim has a history of heart disease.
- If the child is under 12 months old.
- Anytime the gag reflex does not work properly. Examples of this condition are:
  - o If the person is over 65.
  - o If the victim has taken Valium.
  - o If the victim is drunk.
  - o If the person is drowsy.

IN ANY OF THESE CASES CALL A HEALTH PROFESSIONAL IMMEDIATELY IF YOU SUSPECT A POISONING.

SHELF-LIFE

Keep ipecac on hand and replace it every 5 years if you don't use it. If the bottle is opened the product will be effective for 1 year.

Optional Drugs for Symptomatic Relief

ANTI-DIARRHEAL PREPARATIONS

Because diarrhea often helps to clear the body of infection, try to avoid use of an anti-diarrheal for the first 6 hours. Then use only if the diarrhea causes cramping and discomfort.

Anti-diarrheal drugs are of 2 types: those which act to thicken the stool and those which work by slowing the spasm of the intestine which is causing the diarrhea.

The thickening mixtures contain clay or fruit pectin and tend to absorb the bacteria and toxins in the intestine. Although they are safe in that they do not go into the system, they also absorb bacteria needed in digestion. Their continued use is not advised.

Good thickening products are those which contain kaolin (an inactive clay), attapulgite (another clay), or pectin.

Pargel, Kaopectate, and *Kaocon* (concentrated, flavored Kaopectate) contain kaolin and pectin. *Quintess* contains attapulgite.

DOSE

Be sure to give a large enough dose. Anti-diarrheal preparations should be taken following the loose stool until the stool thickens. Then they should be stopped immediately to avoid constipation.

Antispasmodic anti-diarrheal preparations stop the spasm of the intestine. These products contain *paregoric*. Paregoric contains opium and must be used with caution. In many states small amounts of paregoric are available without prescription, but an adult often must sign for it.

Give 1 teaspoon of paregoric in a little fruit juice to an adult or adult-sized child. Give proportionately less to smaller children. Do not give more often than every

4 hours. If it does not work after 2 doses, call a health professional.

Some products contain both thickening and antispasmodic ingredients: two examples are *Donnagel* and *Parepectolin*.

PRECAUTIONS

Do not use products with paregoric for infants under 6 months. They can cause paralysis of the bowel, which can be fatal. For infants age 6 months to 1 year, get advice from a health professional as to dose.

Try the clay products first since they are the safest. When anyone has diarrhea there is a danger of dehydration from loss of body fluids and salts. You should attempt to have the person drink extra liquids after a few hours of giving nothing. Sometimes an electrolytically balanced solution, as shown below, is best.

ASPIRIN AND ACETAMINOPHEN

Aspirin is widely used for relieving pain and reducing fever. It also reduces swelling and inflammation and is valuable for that reason in treating arthritis symptoms. It can also be used to relieve minor itching.

POTENTIAL DANGERS OR SIDE EFFECTS OF ASPIRIN

- More childhood poisonings are caused by aspirin than by any other drug. Three to four grains per pound of body weight is a deadly dose. That's 3–4 baby aspirin per pound a child weighs.
- Aspirin can irritate the stomach lining and occasionally cause stomach bleeding.
- Some people are allergic to aspirin.

Acetaminophen does not seem to have the potential dangers aspirin has. There is less likelihood of allergic reaction, and acetaminophen does not irritate the stomach lining.

However, acetaminophen does *not* reduce swelling or inflammation and is *not* recommended for treatment of arthritis.

Electrolyte Solution for Prevention of Dehydration

- These solutions are electrolytically balanced, similar to the body's fluids.
- Can be purchased from a pharmacist: Pedialyte, Lytren
- Can be purchased at a supermarket: Gatorade
- Can be made at home: 3 oz. water, 1 teaspoon sugar, 1 pinch salt
- Use to replace fluids lost through vomiting, diarrhea, perspiring.

Note: Persons on a low sodium diet should check the contents of these products before using them.

WHEN NOT TO TAKE ASPIRIN

- If suffering from gout
- If taking anticoagulants (blood thinners)
- For a hangover—before or after alcohol. Aspirin, an acid, can irritate the already upset stomach.

SIGNS OF ASPIRIN POISONING (SALICYLISM)

- Ringing in ears
- Rapid, deep breathing
- Visual disturbances
- Nausea
- Dizziness

Discontinue use if any of the above symptoms occur. Call a health professional if rapid, deep breathing, visual disturbances, nausea, or dizziness occurs.

IN CASE OF OVERDOSE

- Call health professional, poison control center, or emergency room.
- Induce vomiting with syrup of ipecac.

BUYING HINTS

When buying aspirin, you need not get the most expensive brands, but sometimes the cheapest aspirin will deteriorate more rapidly than others. If it smells like vinegar, don't buy it.

Additives to aspirin tablets may be useful, but will not be more effective than aspirin in reducing pain. You run less risk of ill effects by taking the simplest drug possible.

Acetaminophen is available under brand names such as *Tylenol, Prompt, Nebs,* and *Datril.* Children's liquid aspirin, such as *Liquiprin,* is actually acetaminophen. Read the label and buy an inexpensive, simple formula.

STORAGE

Aspirin and acetaminophen should be stored in a locked cabinet. Keep dry and cool. Use childproof bottles, if possible. Do not refrigerate.

SHELF-LIFE

- Aspirin: One year. Discard when strong odor of vinegar is present.
- Acetaminophen: Two years.

COLD MEDICATIONS

Antibiotics will neither cure a cold nor relieve its symptoms.

Some over-the-counter products may provide temporary relief of cold symptoms but they are not necessary. Use them if they help you feel better or if they help you rest while recovering. Rest and liquids are probably the best treatments for colds.

Dosage for Aspirin and Acetaminophen

ASPIRIN	ACETAMINOPHEN
Adults — 5 grains (1 tablet)	
Children's — 1 ¼ grains (1 tablet)	
Take every 3 - 4 hours, as needed	Take every 3 hours, as needed
1 year — 1 children's	Under 1 year — 0.6cc* (liquid)
2 ½ — 2 children's	1 - 3 — 0.6-1.2 ccs
4 — 3 children's	3 - 6 — 1.2 ccs
5 - 6 — 4 children's or 1 adult	6 - 12 — ½ - 1 tablet
7 - 8 — 1 ½ adult	Adults — 1 - 3 tablets
10 and up — 2 adult	
Adults — 1 - 3 tablets	*All liquid aspirin comes with droppers marked in cubic centimeters (ccs)

Doses are approximate. What is important is to give enough to provide relief. One baby aspirin every 4 hours probably won't reduce a 4-year-old's fever.

Decongestants

Decongestants make breathing easier by shrinking the swollen mucous membranes of the nose and allowing air to pass through the nose. Decongestants also help relieve a runny nose and provide some relief for postnasal drip, which can cause a sore throat. In some cases early use of oral decongestants during a cold will prevent the eustachian tube from swelling and prevent ear infections.

Decongestants can be taken orally, or as nose drops, or as sprays. Oral decongestants are distributed through the bloodstream, are probably more effective, and last longer. Sprays and drops provide immediate, temporary relief. Measurement of dose is easier with drops.

Sudafed is a good over-the-counter oral decongestant. *Do not* give to infants under 1 year of age.

Neo-synephrine and *Biomydrin* (¼ %-adults, ⅛ %-children) are effective nasal solutions for temporary relief.

PRECAUTIONS

Decongestants can cause drowsiness in some people or increased activity in others.

Medicated nasal sprays or drops should not be used more than 3 days nor more than 3 times a day. With continued use of nose drops a kind of addiction to the drops known as the "rebound" effect may occur. The mucous membranes swell as in a cold. This can also cause loss of sense of smell.

The safest nasal drop for stuffy nose is a saline solution made at home. Saline nose drops will not cause a rebound effect. They provide comfort by keeping nasal tissues moist so they can work to filter the air. Saline nose drops are also okay to use on infants with a stuffy nose. Put in drops, then suck out the mucus with a bulb aspirator.

STORAGE

Most non-prescription tablets and capsules will last 1 year if stored in a cool, dry place. Nasal decongestant drops and sprays are generally good for up to 1 year.

Try to prevent the dropper from touching the nose.

Antihistamines

Antihistamines were originally developed to treat the symptoms of allergy. They are now included in most products for cold relief, in combination with a decongestant. By drying up the mucous membranes, antihistamines make the person more comfortable, whether the problem is a cold or an allergy.

Many cold preparations such as *Dristan, Coricidin,* and *Triaminic* contain both decongestants and antihistamines. *Novahistine* is safe for young children. *Chlor-Trimetron* is available over-the-counter as a pure antihistamine. Do *not* use antihistamines for children under 4 months. For children aged 4 months to 1 year obtain a health professional's advice regarding correct dose.

Antihistamines are occasionally used to relieve itching and to relieve motion sickness if *Drama-*

Saline Nose Drops

¼ teaspoon salt in 1 cup distilled water (too much salt will dehydrate nasal membranes).

Place in a clean bottle with dropper (available at drugstore). Place drops in affected nose as frequently as necessary. Discard and make a fresh solution weekly.

Inserting Drops: Have patient lie down, head hanging over the side of the bed. In this way the drops get farthest back.

mine or *Marezine* are not available. A product containing only antihistamines, without added decongestants, is best.

PRECAUTIONS

The value of antihistamines in treating cold symptoms has not been proven. Some health professionals believe that by drying the mucous membranes antihistamines may prolong a cold. Moist membranes are needed to filter infection. Remember these products dry *all* mucous membranes. Drink extra fluids when taking cold medications. Antihistamines can cause drowsiness or increased activity, depending on the individual.

BUYING HINTS

Ask your pharmacist for a suitable product then read the label. Often more ingredients mean simply more money, not more effectiveness. Time-release capsules can be more convenient, but they may also be more expensive.

STORAGE

Store in cool, dry place. Shelf-life: 1 year.

Cough Preparations

Coughing is the body's method of expelling foreign substances and phlegm or mucus from the respiratory tract. Therefore, coughs are often useful and you usually don't want to eliminate them. Occasionally, however, they are severe enough to impair breathing or prevent rest.

Water and other liquids, such as fruit juices, are probably the best cough "syrup." They moisten, soothe, and thin mucus so it can be coughed up more easily. Any increase in fluid intake will also help thin secretions.

There are 2 kinds of cough preparations. The first, *expectorants,* help to thin the mucus, making it easier to "get it up." *Romilar* and *Robitussin* are good expectorant cough syrups. Look for those containing glyceryl guaiacolate.

The second kind of cough preparation is used to control or suppress a nagging cough. These are called *suppressants*. They actually suppress the cough reflex. These are for the dry, nagging, hacking cough that won't let you rest. Dextromethorphan is a good ingredient to look for in suppressant cough preparations. *Cheracol-D* and *Dorcol* are effective.

PRECAUTIONS

If a cough persists for more than 5 days, you should at least call a health professional.

Suppressant cough syrups work by suppressing the cough reflex. They can also suppress breathing and should be used with caution, especially with young children. Suppressants should not be used if the person has a constipation problem.

Many cough preparations also contain ingredients for relief of other cold symptoms and several contain a large percent of alcohol. Read the labels so you know what ingredients you are taking. It can be a waste of money and is potentially harmful to take decongestants in several forms. There are many choices. Your pharmacist can advise you.

The simplest *cough syrup* often can be made at home. It soothes irritated throat tissue. Mix 1 part lemon juice and 2 parts honey. This can be given in ¼ teaspoon doses even to small infants.

Cough drops are largely ineffective. The melting drops can soothe the throat, but so will water. Candy cough drops are just as effective as medicated over-the-counter drops. Cough drops are not advised for children under 6, however, as they can go into the windpipe and cause choking.

Laxatives

Laxatives are widely overused by Americans. Probably only 1 child in 100 needs a laxative. For guidelines, see Constipation on page 29. Even in adults the use of laxatives often creates more problems than it solves.

A laxative is defined as any compound which eases the passage and elimination of feces (bowel movement). Water is the simplest and best laxative. Increasing fluid intake is the first treatment to try for constipation. Also, increasing your roughage intake (bran, lettuce, leafy vegetables, fruits such as prunes, apples) may provide relief. Often simply increasing your activity level will stimulate bowel movement. If these natural remedies do not work, try the following preparations.

For infants: Add *Maltsupex* to the formula or give in a bottle. It is safe, not habit-forming and it acts as a stool softener. However, laxatives are *rarely* needed for infants and you should investigate the possible causes before trying any commercial remedy.

For children and adults: Mineral oil is a good lubricant. Do not force it down a child. If inhaled into the lungs, mineral oil can cause a type of pneumonia. Do not use regularly. Mineral oil slows the body's absorption of vitamins A, D, E, and K. Also, it can "leak" out the anus and be inconvenient.

Colace is a stool softener safe for children.

Peri-colace acts as a stimulant to get digestive waves moving and force contents of intestines on through the digestive tract and to soften the stool.

PRECAUTIONS

No laxative should be taken if there is abdominal pain. If the problem is appendicitis, the stimulation of a laxative could rupture the appendix.

Do not take laxatives regularly. The regular use of laxatives decreases tone and sensation of the large intestine and develops dependency on the laxative.

Increase water intake when taking any laxative.

Miscellaneous Medications

ANTIBIOTICS

Antibiotics are drugs that kill certain harmful bacteria which cause disease. There are many different types of antibiotics, all of which are produced naturally by micro-organisms. By killing bacteria and limiting their multiplication, the antibiotics allow your own infection fighting system to cure you of an infection.

Generally, antibiotics stop the synthesis of protein in the cell wall of a bacterium. The bacteria die without this protein cell wall. However, antibiotics are only effective against bacteria; they have no effect on a virus. Therefore, *antibiotics have no use in curing the common cold* or any other virus-caused illness.

There are many different kinds of bacteria; some are helpful in our bodies, some are harmless, and some cause diseases. Different antibiotics attack different bacteria. Penicillin works against some bacteria, tetracycline against others. Ampicillin is a "broad spectrum antibiotic;" it kills many different types of bacteria, but it is closely related to penicillin.

An antibiotic will kill all the bacteria in the body which are sensitive to it—whether they are harmful or helpful. Thus, the balance in your body may be destroyed while you are taking an antibiotic and you may develop stomach upset, a vaginal infection, or some other problem. That is one potential *side effect* (something that happens besides the intended effect of a drug) of antibiotics. This side effect can sometimes be prevented by using Bacid (a capsule of helpful bacteria) or, more simply, by eating yogurt or buttermilk, foods which stimulate the growth of healthful bacteria.

You should take antibiotics only when needed to fight a *bacterial* infection. There are several reasons for this:

First, antibiotics can cause many side effects, most mild, some very severe. People react differently to drugs. If at *any* time you have *any* unexpected reaction to an antibiotic, tell your health professional *before* any other antibiotic is prescribed.

Second, bacteria build resistance to antibiotics. Taken too frequently, an antibiotic may be less effective. The indiscriminate use of antibiotics in some countries has already rendered some antibiotics useless.

Third, some people are allergic to antibiotics and may experience severe, life-threatening reactions.

Fourth, if the antibiotic is not useful in fighting the infection, why waste your time, money, energy, and health?

When you and your health professional have decided that an antibiotic is necessary and you have a prescription, follow the instructions accurately.

Take the whole dose for as many days as prescribed. Ask your health professional how long you should take the prescription. Antibiotics kill off many of the harmful bacteria quite quickly, so you are apt to feel better in a few days. You *must* continue to take the medication so it can continue to kill the bacteria until your body can control the infection. If you stop too soon, it is likely that only the weaker bacteria have been eliminated and that the stronger ones will survive and flourish. You may well become even sicker in a few days.

Unless there are severe unexpected side effects continue the dose for the full time prescribed.

When taking an antibiotic, as any medication, you must follow instructions carefully. Taking a capsule with meals or an hour before can mean all the difference in effectiveness of certain antibiotics. Be sure you understand any special instructions about taking the medication. These *should* be on the bottle label, but ask your physician and your pharmacist if there are special instructions about taking an antibiotic. For example, some antibiotics are ineffective if taken with alcohol. Alcohol stimulates the kidneys to quickly expel more fluid than that taken in as alcohol, so some of the antibiotic will leave the body prematurely. Also, an irritated stomach lining will not absorb the medication as well.

Page 229 lists many antibiotics and precautions for their use.

STORAGE

As far as storage of antibiotics, pills and tablets should be stored in a dry, cool place. They will usually keep their potency for about a year. However, most are prescribed only for a specific illness in an amount to be completed during that illness. *NEVER* give an antibiotic prescribed for one person to another. Do not take an antibiotic for another illness without a health professional's instructions.

Liquid antibiotics are always dated; most are good for 2 weeks if refrigerated, for 1 if kept at room temperature.

VITAMINS

With the exception of infants, and pregnant women and nursing mothers, few people need vitamin supplements. A reasonably well-balanced diet usually provides more than enough of the vitamins and other nutrients the body needs to thrive. Sometimes some minerals

Antibiotic Advice

elow is a list of commonly prescribed antibiotic drugs. Your physician should tell you when and with what
oods to take a prescription, but if not, and you have forgotten to ask, refer to this chart. By following these
structions, you will ensure that your prescription is most effective.

ANTIBIOTIC	One hour before or two hours after meals	On empty stomach but food may lessen upset	With meals	After meals	Not with milk or antacids	Not with antacids	Not with fruit juices	Food may ease gastric upset
DYNAPEN	X							
LINCOCIN	X							
PATHOCIL	X							
PENICILLIN G	X							
PROSTHAPHLIN	X							
RONDOMYCIN	X				X			
UNIPEN	X							
VERACILLIN	X							
TEGOPEN	X							
VERSAPEN	X							
TETRACYCLINES	X				X		X	X
Achromycin								
Mysteclin								
Panmycin								
Symycin								
Tetracyn								
Tetrex								
Declomycin								
Etc.								
TAO		X						
KEFLEX	X							
AMPICILLIN	X							X
VIBRAMYCIN			X			X	X	
ERYTHROMYCIN								
Ilosone		X						
E - Mycin	X							X
Erythrocin	X							X
PENICILLIN VK			X					
CLEOCIN			X					
BETAPEN VK			X					
VEETIDS			X					

are lacking, such as iron, and your health professional may suggest a supplement. Iron supplements may cause bowel movements to appear black, almost tarry. Also, fluoride supplements, available by prescription only, may be given to young children as a decay prevent-ative. Many people, however, routinely use vitamin supplements for their families "just to be on the safe side."

Aside from the unnecessary expense, there can be in some cases a good deal of danger in giving extra, un-needed vitamins. The body gen-

General Purpose, Useful Medications

PRODUCT	BRAND NAME	PURPOSE	STORAGE	SHELF-LIFE
Hydrogen Peroxide		Minor cuts, abrasions; mouth-wash (diluted)	Cool, dry, locked	One year + (as long as bubbles appear when applied to wound)
Petrolatum (solid mineral oil) petroleum jelly	Vaseline	Dry skin; to repel water (diaper rash); minor abrasions, burns	Anywhere	Indefinitely. Gets rancid if too old
Antibiotic Creams	Neosporin Mycitracin	Abrasions, skin infections	Cool, dry place	Tube will be dated, up to 4 years
Antiseptic Cream	First Aid Cream	Abrasions, cuts	Cool, dry place	Indefinitely
Rubbing Alcohol 70%		Antiseptic; clean thermometer	Tightly closed	Indefinitely

erally expels whatever extra vitamins it cannot use with no known harm. But some vitamins (A, D, E, and K) are stored by the body until needed and if too many are taken, vitamin overdose and serious illness can result. It is generally not advisable to take vitamin supplements except when recommended by a health professional.

GENERAL PURPOSE, USEFUL MEDICATIONS

The table above charts several medications you may wish to keep in your home health center. They are convenient for occasional use and have been found through experience to be effective. Remember that soap and water is your best cleaning product.

15

Family Medical Records

One important way to accept responsibility for your family's health is by maintaining precise, up-to-date family medical records. Good accurate home records will guide your self-care decisions when future problems arise. They will also be of help to health professionals in diagnosing more complex problems that might arise. Most of all, good records will allow you to learn from past experiences and will help build your confidence and ability to care for similar problems in the future.

This book contains examples of medical records for your family. You could buy a 3-ring binder with blank pages to write your own records. Use the forms provided here as a guide for making yours. All family members should have separate sets of records so when they leave home, they can each have their own records.

In addition to the forms you make from the ones provided, you may already have information on each family member. If possible, add that information to your notebook. It is best to have all information in one place regardless of the form. You should try to gather all data on each family member now, even if they are almost grown. They still need to know which immunizations they have had, to which drugs or substances they are allergic, and from what cause their relatives died.

Following is a discussion of each of the forms in order of appearance. Refer to the discussion if you have difficulty completing any of the forms.

Emergency Telephone Numbers

Make a form such as the one shown for easy reference. Tape it inside your phone book or place it beside your telephone. Names and employers of you and your spouse are listed for a babysitter to use in an emergency.

Drug Inventory

Each time you purchase a drug, whether by prescription or over-the-counter, record the drug name, date of purchase, etc., in the appropriate column. Periodically glance at the record and discard and replace any out-of-date drugs. This form will have most value if you write down every drug or medication used. That way, any possible ill effects from drug interaction can be quickly traced. The last column is reserved for listing any adverse reactions to the drug (ADR), whether you think it worked well or poorly, and other general comments.

Record of Health Professionals

Occasionally, your present health professional may wish to confer with health professionals you visited in the past. This form, properly completed, would then be useful.

Birth Information

The information recorded on this form will be needed when your child enters school and will be use-

ful for a new health professional should you change.

Family History

Many diseases are hereditary. If you have a complete family history of all blood relatives, then your health professional may more easily diagnose a particular disease that you have. You will also be able to see trends in your family tree towards certain ailments that you may be able to avoid. For example, if a number of your grandparents, aunts, and uncles died of heart diseases at an early age, you should consider that you have a high risk for an attack and take appropriate precautions.

At first glance, it may seem unnecessary to fill out this form for each family member. But remember, each child needs a form when he or she leaves home.

Record of Immunizations

Everyone should take advantage of the protection against serious diseases immunizations provide. Sadly, in recent years, there has been an increase in polio and measles because parents aren't having their children immunized. The following immunization schedule should be followed to insure your child against contracting the disease.

Immunization Schedule

Age	DTP	Polio	DT	Measles	Rubella	Mumps
2 months	X	X				
4 months	X	X				
6 months	X	X				
After 15 months				X	X	X
18 months	X	X				
5 years	X	X				
Every 8 - 10 years			X			

REACTION

Reaction to immunizations should be recorded. It is not unusual for a baby to have a fever of 102–103 degrees 2–4 hours after injection. The temperature should return to normal after 24 hours. Also, the leg or arm may be red, swollen, or hard where the injection was given. If the reaction seems to be excessive, tell your health professional and perhaps the next injection can be divided into 2–3 parts and given at 2–3 day intervals to lessen the reaction.

DIPHTHERIA, TETANUS, AND PERTUSSIS (DTP)

DTP is an immunization for diphtheria, tetanus, and pertussis, or whooping cough. This immunization is given as a series of 3 injections beginning at 1–2 months of age. They are spaced at 1–2 month intervals until all 3 injections are given. Boosters for diphtheria and tetanus (DT) are recommended every 8–10 years. The first one would be given at age 15. The part of the immunization for whooping cough is eliminated after 5 years of age, because the disease is not fatal after infancy and reactions to the immunization increase with age.

Tetanus is a bacterial infection that can be fatal. The germ enters the body through cuts and thrives only in the absence of oxygen. So the deeper and narrower the wound, the greater the possibility of tetanus. Tetanus not only occurs from a rusty nail wound or animal bite but can also occur from flying objects from lawn mowers and innocent scratches from boards, rocks, and metal. Once the tetanus infection does occur, the victim has only a 50% chance of survival. Since it is sometimes very difficult to tell if a wound is contaminated with tetanus, the only sure protection is immunization.

There are 2 types of immunization, active or toxoid and passive or antitoxin. Active immunization is achieved by a basic series of 3 shots followed by a booster a year later. Routine boosters are then recommended every 8–10 years to keep the immunized state active. If you have maintained this schedule for tetanus shots, then there is no need for additional boosters unless you have a wound that may be contaminated. In the case of contamination you should get another shot if you haven't had one in the past *5 years*. This is a recent recommendation. A few years ago you received a shot for a wound if you had not had one in the past year.

If you have never been immunized against tetanus, then a passive immunization will be given if you receive a contaminated wound. This shot is first given to cover the situation until active immunization can be developed. These shots may give occasional severe local reactions but only very rarely do they cause serious generalized reactions. At the same time this shot is given, a series of 3 immunization shots is started. The other 2 shots must be given during the next several months.

If you have never been immunized against tetanus, it is a good idea to start the series of 3 active shots now, then have a booster every 8–10 years. You will then be protected against tetanus in the event of a contaminated wound. Keep a record of tetanus boosters received so it is readily available should you be injured.

POLIO

Polio vaccine is given to prevent polio, also known as infantile paralysis. This vaccine is given in 3 successive intervals and boosters are given at 18 months and at 5 years. This vaccine is not recommended for adults as it can cause a serious reaction. A few years ago, polio was a common disease. Now it can be prevented if parents will simply have their children immunized. Polio has not been eliminated as a disease in this country and there has been an increase in cases lately because of lack of immunization.

The Salk vaccine is a dead virus and was given in the form of a shot; it is not used today. The more effective Sabin vaccine is a live virus that is administered orally. Indicate which vaccine was given on the immunization form.

MEASLES, MUMPS, AND RUBELLA

MMR is an immunization for measles, mumps, and Rubella. It is now available as one shot although a few years ago each disease was immunized against separately. Room has been left on the form for you to record whichever way the immunizations were received.

It is important to immunize against a seemingly mild disease as measles (also called rubeola, red measles, or regular measles) as it can lead to complications such as ear infections, pneumonia, encephalitis, or even brain damage. In the 1960s, the measles vaccine was made with a dead virus. It has since been discovered that this particular vaccine doesn't provide lifelong immunity. A new measles vaccine, made from a live virus, is available. If you were given the dead virus vaccine you received an additional shot of gamma globulin. If you had the old vaccine you should be re-immunized.

Mumps is another disease you should be immunized against because of its complications. It can lead to encephalitis, nerve deafness, and sterility in males after puberty. Adult males who have never had mumps should be immunized. Female adults should also be immunized since mumps can go to the ovaries which is very painful.

It is important to immunize against Rubella (also called German, soft, or mild measles) because it causes severe damage to the unborn child if a pregnant woman gets the disease in the first 3 months of pregnancy. All children should be immunized against this disease to prevent a pregnant woman from contracting it. If a woman plans to become pregnant, she should check her family medical records to see if she has had Rubella or the immunization. If not, she can be tested by her health professional to determine this. If it is discovered that she has not had either the disease or the immunization, then she should be immunized. Sometimes, however, health professionals are reluctant to give the immunization because the woman should absolutely not get pregnant in the following 3 months while the vaccine is in her system. This should be discussed with the health professional.

OTHERS

This space is for those who have had immunizations some years ago that are not recommended today. One example is the smallpox vaccination. There has not been a reported case of smallpox in the United States since 1949, but there have been cases of sickness and even death from the vaccine. So unless you plan to travel outside the United States, and even then to only a few countries where the disease is not yet completely controlled, you will not need this vaccination. Your health professional will be able to determine if you need this vaccination after being told which country you will be visiting.

This section could also be used to record up-dated immunizations. An example is the live-virus measles vaccine.

TUBERCULIN TESTS

A tuberculin test is not really an immunization, but rather a skin test for tuberculosis. A positive result does not necessarily mean that you have tuberculosis, but rather that the germ has entered the body.

Usually your body defense mechanism will successfully combat the infection. If you have a positive reaction, then an annual chest X-ray may be advisable. Once a person has a positive reaction to a tuberculin test, the test should not be repeated. You will always have a positive reaction. Subsequent skin tests may cause more severe reactions. This test should be done late in the first year of life prior to the MMR, then done periodically. Your health professional will determine how often tests are needed depending on the prevalence of tuberculosis in your area.

Record of Illnesses, Accidents, and Surgeries

Keep a record of illnesses to help your family. You may recognize that your child has an abnormal number of "colds" each year and suspect an allergy. Records of accidents and surgeries can be useful for insurance purposes. Comments can include any home treatment given, days administered, and name of health professional, if consulted.

Dental Records

If this form is kept up-to-date you can readily see when you last had your teeth checked or cleaned to determine your next appointment. It will also be useful to see if you are having more fillings, in which case you would want to start flossing and brushing more regularly.

Home Physical Exam

This form has been explained in detail beginning on page 4.

Emergency Telephone Numbers

Ambulance _____   Poison Control Center _____

Hospital _____   Police _____

Fire _____   Taxi _____

Mental Health Emergency _____

Doctor _____   Name _____

Friend/ Relative _____   Name _____

	Name	Telephone	Employer
Wife			
Husband			

Drug Inventory

DRUG	PURPOSE/PERSON	RX NO.	COST	INSTRUCTIONS	DATE PURCH.	EXPIR. DATE	POSSIBLE SIDE EFFECTS	USE EFFECT Adverse Drug Reaction (if any)

RECORD OF HEALTH PROFESSIONALS

Health Professional's Name and Address	Specialty	Office Phone and Hours	Dates Started and Ended	Comments

BIRTH INFORMATION

Name _____

Date of Birth _____ Length _____

Time of Birth _____ Weight _____

Blood Type _____

Type of Feeding _____

Name of Hospital _____

    and Address _____

_____

_____

Name of Physician _____

    and Address _____

_____

_____

Details of birth [include details such as duration of pregnancy, length of labor, Caesarean delivery, use of forceps, newborn respiratory distress, jaundice, or birth defects]

_____

_____

_____

_____

_____

_____

_____

_____

_____

Family History

Name _____

Names of Family Members	If Deceased, Age and Cause	Diseases such as diabetes, heart disease, cancer, allergies, hypertension, alcoholism, ulcers, stroke, mental illness, epilepsy, etc.
Great-Grandparents		
Grand Parents		
Aunts and Uncles		
Parents		
Brothers and Sisters		
Children		

Record of Immunizations

Name _____

Test		Date Given	Reaction	Test	Date Given	Reaction
Diphtheria/ Tetanus/ Pertussis or DTP Boosters	First Second Third 18 months 5 years			MMR or Measles Mumps Rubella		
Tetanus Boosters (every 8 - 10 years)				Others		
Polio	First Second Third			Tuberculin Tests		
Boosters	18 months 5 years					

RECORD OF ILLNESSES,
ACCIDENTS AND SURGERIES

Name _____

Date	Description	Health Professional	Comments

DENTAL RECORD

Name _____

Date	Name of Professional	Comments

HOME PHYSICAL EXAM

Date _____. Name _____

Time of day _____

VITAL SIGNS

Height	Weight

Temperature
    Rectal   Oral
	Pulse
	    Beats per minute? Regular?

Respiration Breaths per minute?	Blood Pressure

Reason for physical exam _____

Overall impression, comments _____

Mental health observations _____

Skin	Skull, hair, scalp
Eyes Pupil constriction:	Nose
Ears Hearing	Mouth, teeth

HOME PHYSICAL EXAM
(Continued)

Throat	Neck, lymph nodes
	Chin to chest:
Chest, breasts	Spine
Abdomen	Genitals
Anus Bowel movements	Legs and arms
Hands, nails	Feet, nails
Chest, lungs, heart sounds	Infants (under 2)
Adult women (over 18) Breast	

Additional comments: _____

_____

_____

Index